Yoga for Seniors Ages 50-70

Step by Step Guidebook to Yoga Exercises that are Perfectly Designed for Seniors

By

David F. Thorsen

The Star Publications

About the Author

David F. Thorsen is a famous yoga teacher. He is an expert in teaching the senior community and has a vibrant personality. He has the energy and true passion for his teachings and always wants to inspire and motivate all the old people around him.

He has written this book to impart his skills to those who are unable to move out of their house and want to learn yoga right in the comfort of their homes. He is currently working in a famous Yoga studio as a Lead Trainer and is a passionate supporter of modern technologies who believes in physical activity as the sole way of resolving the problems of the mind and body. He also believes in eating healthy and has always preached health as the biggest wealth.

Download Your Free Gift

Thank you for purchasing this book and we hope you find it useful. Please consider leaving an honest review online check out some of our other publications using the link below:

thestarpublications.com

In order to express our **"gratitude"** to you for purchasing our book, we have a free gift for you:

"Secrets to Keeping and Strengthening Your Marriage"

Visit the link below to grab your free copy:

thestarpublications.com/#get-a-free-book

If you have any **query**, please feel free to write us at:

info@thestarpublications.com

Table of Contents

Introduction

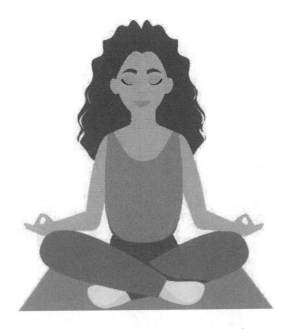

What if you come to know that all the thoughts you had about your mental and physical health after 50 were a paradox? All the time you spent creating those little "easy to handle" moments in your head were just not TRUE? Everything you were telling yourself about health was WRONG all this time?

We live in an era of technology and science. Every day we get to know about something unique and amazing. Still, in this modern era, we are unable to find happiness easily. I have met so many people of different age groups who brag about the sadness in their lives. Many even blamed it on the lockdown sessions we had due to COVID-19. Well, I have thought a lot about these different situations of various people around me and have come to one simple conclusion. It is all in our heads!

Why have we suddenly stopped looking for the silver lining in different circumstances of life? In short, it is the perspective that we need to change and not the people or the situations. I started practicing yoga and taking care of my dietetic routine when I was in my early twenties, and it was a life-changer for me. Before changing my exercise and eating routine, I was going through a lot of mental stress and used to sleep all day long to avoid my problems. A friend of mine suggested yoga when she got to know about my distressful condition and I am happy to say my life has been stress-free ever since I started yoga. I feel like I have been reborn into a completely different individual.

Happiness is a form of energy that starts from the core of our hearts. It is we who need fixing and not just others or our situations. I can understand how you are feeling right now because I have gone through the same feelings in the past. I know you wake up in the morning and feel like you have lost everything. You feel like a complete loser, and I just want to tell you that it is okay not to feel "okay" sometimes. Your body is in pain, and you just feel lost. It is okay to lose yourself because that is when you start finding yourself. Age is just a number, and you need to stop thinking about your age and start focusing on the person you are.

Let's get to the fun part because it is time to say goodbye to all your miseries! You do not have to waste your time and money on any health and fitness programs anymore because now you can get fit and improve your health at home. It is time to relax and feel happy all over again. You can be in the comfort of your home and see yourself grow into a satisfied and positive individual. No more annoying behavior and unhappy thoughts to think about. I promise you that after reading this book, you will have a changed perspective not only about life but also about yourself. You will fall in love with the inner strength and calmness in your body that you gain after every yoga session and a healthy meal.

This book will help you learn all the exciting details you need to know about health and fitness. You will learn the different advantages of yoga and will understand how yoga can change the course of your life forever. Through this book, you will learn everything from healthy body mechanics to what your body needs once you reach the age of 50, and acquire the skill of keeping yourself motivated for yoga sessions every day. This book will also give you some amazing insights about your eating routine, a one-week diet plan, and how you can improve the standard of your life with healthy eating habits. I will walk you through, step by step, until you have mastered everything necessary to achieve your desired goals.

Getting to know yourself completely is the first step towards a satisfied and happy life. Keep reading if you want to relieve stress, have a healthy workout, and plant the seeds of health and strength in your body. I am sure you will enjoy this book.

Chapter 1: Yoga - The Solution to All Your Health Problems

I am sure that when you hear the word 'yoga,' a picture of an individual curving in an excruciating yoga act springs up in your mind. Indeed, all the "Asanas" or yoga poses are challenging to do initially and would surely scare anyone who is new to yoga. Yet, yoga poses are not that scary once you start practicing them regularly. So, I would like to ask you how well you truly know yoga? The world consistently observes Yoga's International Day in June every year, so how about if we disentangle the secrets of this beautiful concept that began in India?

Yoga is an old activity that focuses on improving strength, adaptability, flexibility, and breathing to support mental and physical prosperity. The principal parts of yoga are different Asanas (poses) and chakras (energy centers). These Asanas and chakras are a progression of development intended to build strength and adaptability in the human body. Yoga, which originated in India approximately five millennia ago, has undergone several adaptations in various countries worldwide. Yoga is ubiquitous in recreational communities, fitness centers, schools, and emergency clinics and is also used for multiple medical procedures.

Over 90% of individuals who start practicing yoga actually perform it to exercise, develop their health, or reduce stress. One research on yoga has discovered that 66% of people who practice yoga have a change in their perspective regarding why they practice yoga regularly. After practicing yoga, people start focusing on self-completion, a feeling of satisfying one's latent capacity. The act of yoga offers definitely more than just poses and headstands. The most important benefits yoga offers are a sense of self-reflection, the act of graciousness and sympathy followed by development, and positive consciousness of yourself and the others around you.

Yoga does not adhere to a specific religion, thought process, or ethnic area. It has forever been drawn closer as a tool for internal prosperity. Any individual who practices yoga regularly can receive its rewards, regardless of age, gender, or culture. Moreover, yoga is usually perceived as a treatment or exercise for well-being and wellness. While physical and emotional wellness is an obvious result of yoga, the objective of yoga is much larger. Yoga is tied in with fitting oneself with the rhythm of the universe. It helps people change their life by adjusting their control to the universe's rhythm. This helps them in accomplishing the most significant level of discernment and congruity in life.

With this knowledge in mind, it is an ideal opportunity for you to take your exercise mats out and enjoy the mix of mental and physical tasks that have indulged numerous yoga specialists for centuries. The gloriousness of yoga is that you do not need to be a yoga master to benefit from it. Whether you are old, fit, or overweight, you can calm your mind and induce the magic of serenity in your body through yoga. Yoga supports and benefits all; so, it does not matter if you are over 50, you can start practicing it today. Surely, you will fall in love with the magic of yoga with the help of this chapter, which highlights how important yoga is to your body after the age of 50. Keep reading!

1.1 Your Life without Yoga

Would you be able to envision a world without yoga? It would be similar to a life without many prominent delights such as green smoothies or having a sunbath by the beach. What would you opt for as a relaxing activity in this unnerving imaginary world if yoga did not exist? It would be like living in a box under the stairs. Feels bad, right?

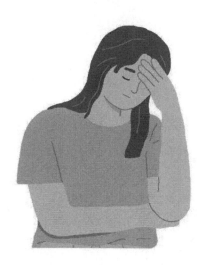

So now, I am sure you would want to know more about yoga and add it to your life because actions start with knowledge. Every single person who practices yoga has achieved the influential power of yoga. Through yoga, many individuals have experienced huge changes in their associations and relationships and point of view in life that helps them feel better in their bodies. However, since these changes routinely happen, it can sometimes be hard to pinpoint unequivocally what it is about yoga that helps you live a happy life.

If one truly wants to understand why yoga is so meaningful, one needs to fathom the changes that yoga will bring into their life. The likelihood that yoga changes you into someone better than the one you were before is something confusing. It is more straightforward to say that yoga helps you take out the impediments that make your genuine personality dull and helps you to come into the true form of your soul. With yoga, you are not just changing into someone you want to be; you are changing into the very person you normally are, that is your best self.

Yoga helps you by negating the negative impact of the changes you have made to your daily chores, especially those that have been made over a long time. When you put your body into a new posture and stay in it for five to ten minutes, you discover many different things about yourself. Taking this new position with your body can lead you to relax and clear out any negative thoughts in your mind. Yoga Asanas isolate the psychological, energetic, physical, vibrant, and spiritualist blocks of life that quell us from thriving when practiced accurately and regularly with attention.

Yoga also helps you in learning how to settle on better choices. Everything about practicing yoga has an aim; when you practice yoga, you start living your life in a very disciplined way. In this way, you focus only on a single goal in life. When you are careful and conscious in your yoga practice, you get the freedom to be more careful and focused in your life.

When you have practiced sincerely, felt completely present, and associated with your body towards the end of yoga practice, you experience a feeling of bliss that is a statement of your real essence. Even though the feeling can be short-lived, it shows that achieving that feeling is possible.

Always remember that only a cheerful and relaxed brain is better positioned to adapt and solve different issues and challenges in life. Yoga keeps the mind serene and content, thus reinforcing your bonds with other individuals. With everyday practice, you become less and less worried and have a better connection between your body and mind even after 50. When you practice yoga, you become better at recognizing how you feel and understanding yourself and your body. Yoga further develops your strengths and resilience. The different poses of yoga strengthen your organs and reinforce your body's muscles while the breathing strategies of yoga remove disagreeableness and anxiety that manifest in your body as afflictions. All of these changes are more needed after we turn 50. So, after knowing all this, do you still not want yoga in your life? If your answer is still "No.", I will take you even deeper into the world of yoga therapy that will surely convince you to practice yoga today. Stay tuned, readers!

1.2 What is Yoga and How Can it Help You?

Yoga is a journey of finding your actual self. If it were just a physical practice or a workout session, you would not be able to find your true self through it. If it were simply an act for entertainment, it might not be as amazing as it is. And, most importantly, you do not need just entertainment after you have turned 50. Strength, fitness, and happiness are what you need the most!

Yoga fundamentally implies something that takes you to your present reality. From a genuine perspective, it focuses mainly on "associations." Association means it takes you to an authoritative reality, where the different appearances of individuals in your life are very clear. Yoga portrays association not as a suspected thought but as a perspective or a thought that you absorb.

It is appropriately said that if a person wants to keep a congruity between oneself and the world, then yoga is best for them. Exercises of yoga have a genuine effect, and they can bring amicability between life's components. Yoga can be practiced at any age; it is healthy for old-age people, requiring no exceptional efforts or adjustments. Yoga helps individuals refine self-thought and self-affirmation through specific thinking, perseverance, discipline, right bearing, benevolence, and humbleness.

Yoga's delicate movements are the reasons behind its popularity and it is great for individuals who have not been very active in some time. Well, consider yourself in the category too because definitely, 50 is usually a low-movement age. It is great for individuals with specific medical issues like joint pain or osteoporosis and can be an extraordinary option if you are unfit and need an activity to keep yourself fit since yoga activities can be changed to meet your requirements. As you become stronger and more experienced with yoga, it becomes easier to perform different sorts of activities like moving, strolling, or swimming even after 50.

Yoga can assist you in staying fit for longer and forestalling back pain and joint injury. It will give you independence and confidence. Moreover, one of the main advantages of any yoga routine is that its benefits stretch across both the physical and the mental aspects of one's life. The main challenge is figuring out how to focus, which can be done by adjusting your consideration, starting from the body and moving to the mind. As you stick with your training over the long term, you begin to see the spiritual and psychological advantages of yoga even after 50.

1.3 Benefits of Practicing Yoga Every Day

If you are an enthusiastic yoga professional, you would have most likely already seen the advantages of yoga. Perhaps you now sleep better, get fewer colds, or simply feel more satisfied and relaxed in life. However, if you are new to yoga and do not know its advantages, then this section is specially written for you. As it occurs, scientific research is beginning to give substantial evidence on how yoga helps one in getting fit, repairing any pain in the body, and keeping any disorder under control, which coupled with my years of experience in yoga and detailed personal research, has brought me to this point that I am writing down all the essential benefits you will get from practicing yoga every day after 50.

1. Yoga Develops Muscle Fortitude

Different Asanas require different muscles to stretch and contract to support our bodies in different positions which strengthen our muscles. Solid muscles are very important for staying healthy for a long time. Practicing yoga regularly can help to protect us from age-related joint conditions and alleviate back pain. The gentle exercises involved in yoga improve flexibility, range of motion, and muscle tone, promoting overall health and well-being. By balancing strength with flexibility, we can cultivate a harmonious relationship with our bodies and enjoy vibrant health throughout our lives.

2. Yoga Develops Flexibility

Yoga offers a clear advantage in terms of improving flexibility. It's common to experience limitations in flexibility when starting out with yoga, such as being unable to touch your toes during a backbend. However, assuming you keep practicing, you will see a steady change in your body's flexibility, and, in the long run, you will be able to practice very difficult postures. You will presumably also see all your body pains vanish away slowly.

3. Yoga Prevents the Breakdown of Ligaments and Joints

By consistently engaging in yoga, one is able to move their joints through their complete range of motion which can effectively ward off degeneration and pain caused by neglect and compression of certain ligaments. Joint ligaments require compression to receive fresh nutrients, much like a sponge. Neglected areas of the ligament can wear out over time, leading to exposed bone and damaged cartilage.

4. Yoga Develops An Ideal Posture

The human head is round and heavy, much like a bowling ball. When it is positioned correctly over an erect spine, the neck, and back muscles require less effort to support its movement. However, poor posture can lead to back and neck pain, as well as other muscle and joint issues, which can eventually result in degenerative joint conditions. Fortunately, yoga offers a simple solution to these problems. Regular practice can improve posture, reducing the risk of neck and back pain and promoting overall joint health.

5. Yoga Strengthens Bones

It is considered that the weight-bearing activity strengthens bones which assist in keeping osteoporosis away, something that many yoga poses can help with since they necessitate that you lift your own weight. Moreover, yoga can bring down levels of the chemical cortisol, a stress hormone, which can strengthen the body by keeping the calcium intact in the bones.

6. Yoga Protects the Spine

The spinal discs act as protective cushions between the vertebrae, preventing herniation and compression of nerves. The nerve endings are the main ways the spine gets its nutrients. If you have an even yoga practice with many backbends, forward twists, and turns, you will strengthen your spinal plates and keep them flexible. As discussed earlier, flexibility is a known advantage of Yoga that is particularly important for the well-being of our spine after 50.

7. Yoga Supports Blood Flow

Yoga can enhance blood circulation throughout your body, particularly in the feet region, due to the relaxation techniques you learn. Through improved levels of hemoglobin and red blood cells, which transport oxygen to your cells and tissues, yoga promotes increased oxygen supply to your cells. Also, platelets become less sticky and fewer unhealthy proteins are present in the bloodstream, reducing blood viscosity. This can lower the risk of cardiovascular events such as heart attacks and strokes, as clotting is often the leading cause.

8. Yoga Helps in Reducing Hypertension

You can take help from yoga if you have hypertension. Two investigations of individuals with hypertension showed a 26-point drop in systolic and a 15-point drop in diastolic pulse.

From these investigations, it is clear to see that yoga is here to help with your blood pressure issues after 50.

9. Yoga Increases Heart Rate

Consistent elevation of your heart rate into the high aerobic range through activities like vigorous yoga can lower the risk of developing coronary heart disease and alleviate depression. While not all types of yoga fall under high aerobic activity, Ashtanga or flow-based classes can effectively increase heart rate. Ashtanga is a form of yoga that follows a series of asanas based on eight principles.

10. Yoga Enhances Joyfulness

According to studies, engaging in yoga on a regular basis can elevate the levels of "feel-good" neurotransmitters like serotonin, while also lowering the levels of cortisol, a hormone related to stress, and monoamine oxidase, an enzyme that breaks down neurotransmitters.

11. Yoga Controls Adrenal Glands

The practice of yoga has been shown to lower the levels of cortisol, which the adrenal glands release during times of stress to help the body cope. However, if cortisol levels remain high even after the stressor is gone, it can lead to negative effects. Although short-term spikes in cortisol can enhance long-term memory, chronic elevations can result in memory impairment and detrimental and sustained brain alterations. Studies on rodents have connected high cortisol levels to tendencies for "food-seeking" behavior and greater storage of abdominal fat, which can contribute to an increased risk of weight gain, diabetes, and heart disease.

12. Yoga Brings Down Glucose and Cholesterol Levels

Diabetes and high cholesterol can be serious issues in old age that can be fixed with yoga. Yoga has been shown to reduce glucose and low-density lipoprotein (LDL) cholesterol levels while increasing high-density lipoprotein (HDL) cholesterol. For individuals with diabetes, yoga can lower glucose levels through various mechanisms such as reducing cortisol and adrenaline levels, promoting weight loss, and improving insulin tolerance. By reducing glucose and cholesterol levels, yoga can lower the risk of heart attack, kidney problems, and vision impairment.

13. Yoga Promotes a Healthy Lifestyle

Yoga offers a two-pronged approach to achieving a healthy lifestyle - it encourages physical movement and calorie burn through regular practice, while also inspiring deeper reflection on diet and weight issues. By promoting mindful eating habits, yoga empowers practitioners to adopt a more balanced approach to their diet. But the benefits of yoga extend beyond the physical realm, resonating throughout all aspects of life and contributing to a more holistic, healthy way of living.

14. Yoga Keeps Up with the Sensory System

Yogis who have attained a high level of proficiency can exert extraordinary control over their bodies, thanks to the power of their nervous systems. Scientific research supports the remarkable abilities of these yogis, who have been known to induce unique heart rhythms, generate specific brain waves, and increase the temperature of their hands by as much as 15 degrees Fahrenheit.

15. Yoga Develops Equilibrium and Stability

Yoga is beneficial in promoting proprioception, which pertains to one's ability to recognize the actions of the body and its spatial awareness, leading to better balance. Individuals with bad posture, knee problems, and back pain are often associated with poor proprioception. Regular yoga practice aids in improving proprioception and balance, thereby minimizing the likelihood of falls and injuries.

16. Yoga Prevents Stomach-Related Issues

Pressure or stress can exacerbate ulcers, unhealthy gut conditions, and constipation. So, logically if you stress less, you will experience fewer stomach issues. Yoga can therefore bring down the danger of colon disease by managing and reducing stress.

17. Yoga Improves Lungs Capacity

Yoga practitioners tend to opt for slower and deeper breathing, resulting in a calming and more effective experience. Over a period of one month, a study observed a decrease in the average respiratory rate of yoga practitioners from 13.4 breaths per minute to 7.6. This resulted in improved physical endurance, as well as increased oxygenation in the blood. Additionally, yoga has been shown to improve various aspects of lung function, such as maximum breath volume and exhalation efficiency.

18. Yoga Gives True Serenity

Yoga suppresses the variances of the brain. As such, it dials back the psychological circles of disappointment, lament, outrage, dread, and stress. Stress leads to many medical issues, from headaches and sleeping disorders to lupus, MS, dermatitis, hypertension, and respiratory failures. So, if you figure out how to calm your brain, you will probably live longer and better.

19. Yoga Provides Internal Strength

Yoga has the potential to bring about positive changes in your life. You may notice that after practicing yoga, you naturally begin to adopt healthier habits such as clean eating, exercising, or even quitting smoking without a deliberate effort.

20. Yoga Increases Confidence Levels

Chronic low self-esteem is a common issue that some may turn to medication to cope with, which can exacerbate the problem. Alternatively, practicing yoga can have a positive impact on one's self-esteem and lead to significant improvements.

Normal yoga practice gives fundamentally higher scores of happiness in individuals, and it is not important to be a specialist in yoga to gain benefits from it. It is an unbelievably relaxing activity to take an interest in even after turning 50. Yoga specialists approach different everyday issues with a more settled point of view, so, to genuinely gain these phenomenal advantages, start adding yoga practice into your life today!

1.4 Your Body's Needs after 50

"Health and fitness is not all that matters, yet without health, nothing feels worthy." It is a famous proverb that demonstrates the significance of the well-being of our bodies in our lives. If our well-being is not exceptional, we cannot accomplish our objectives or stay or attain self actualization.

The human body changes with aging, occurring in individual cells and entire organs. These progressions bring about unwanted changes in the working of the body. As cells grow older, their functionality deteriorates and over time, aged cells undergo a natural process of self-elimination known as apoptosis. The maturing of a cell is a trigger for the initiation of apoptosis.

The effectiveness of our organs is dependent on the optimal functioning of their individual cells. However, as the body ages, cells tend to deteriorate and, in some organs like the testicles, ovaries, liver, and kidneys, cell death outpaces cell replacement, leading to a decline in the organ's overall cell count. When the cell count falls below a certain threshold, the affected organ loses its ability to function as it did in youth.

Although most of the body's functions and capabilities remain intact, the decline in organ function can make it difficult for older individuals to handle challenging situations such as physically demanding work, extreme temperature changes, or hormonal fluctuations. This decline could also be caused by medication side effects or overworking of certain organs.

As an aged grown-up, a standard workout (not heavy workouts but easier ones) is one of the main things you can do for your well-being. It can reduce the likelihood of many of the medical conditions that appear when you turn 50. It can also assist your muscles in developing further so you can continue to do your everyday tasks without becoming reliant upon others. Remember, some active work is important for staying fit and healthy, and as you become more active, your health advantages increase too.

Aged grown-ups with persistent conditions ought to know if their conditions support active workouts. When aged grown-ups cannot complete 150 minutes of moderate-force and high-impact exercise in a week due to persistent conditions, they ought to be pretty much as active as their conditions permit.

Retirement years help people take rest. It is usually said that life dials back with age, i.e., we become kids as we grow old. We laugh a lot more and become more sensitive, just like a kid. However, one thing which is different is our activity levels. As we age, our activity levels decrease which can prompt several issues including seizing of joints, wilting of muscles, and even altering of individuals' intellectual capacities. Accordingly, numerous elderly individuals attempt to track down different ways of keeping themselves more active. Alongside conventional strategies, such as planting or strolling, yoga is becoming famous among aged people to stay in shape and happy in their lives.

Starting or keeping a typical exercise routine can be a challenge at every stage of life, and it does not get any less complex as you age. You may feel discouraged because of clinical issues, constant aggravation, or stresses over injuries or falls. In case you have never worked out, you may not know where to begin, or you may accept you are exorbitantly old or sensitive and cannot complete tasks that you could when you were young. Maybe you feel that certain actions are debilitating.

While these may seem like legitimate reasons to tone down and unwind as you age, they are, by a long shot, better inspirations than anything else. Being more active can stimulate your perspective, ease the pressure, help you with managing disease and pain, and further foster your overall feeling of success. Getting the advantages of movement does not have to incorporate challenging activities or visits to the gym. You can gain benefits from adding many other activities to your life, even in little ways. Whatever your age or condition, it is never too late to get your body moving, support your prosperity, and further improve how well you age.

As we grow old, it becomes crucial to incorporate physical activity into our daily routines to maintain a healthy lifestyle. Regular exercise can help seniors feel more energetic and better equipped to manage the discomfort that often comes with aging. This leads to a more independent life where seniors feel safer and more confident. Yoga has been identified as one of the best forms of exercise for seniors. With time, seniors can improve their flexibility, balance, strength, and agility through yoga, which can help enhance their overall resilience and boost their mood. I am sure you would have gained a pool of knowledge regarding yoga for seniors in this chapter, and the best part is that it does not end here. Keep reading to learn more about yoga for the perfectly imperfect body in the next chapter!

Chapter 2: Yoga for the Perfectly Imperfect Body

I always wanted an ideal physique all my life. Luckily, with yoga, I have learned that I do not need to have one! This is not generally as clear as it might sound. Many of my friends come to me so they can have a model-like physique by learning and practicing yoga. I get this on the grounds that before I started practicing yoga, and up until now, I have wanted all of these things myself!

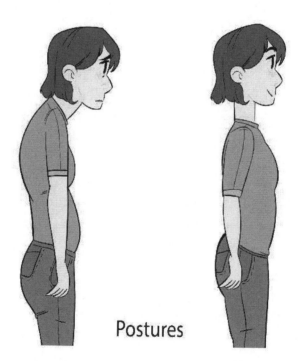

Postures

However, I have found a more impressive and liberating craving inside myself through yoga. Yoga has taught me how to know myself entirely as I truly am. Surprisingly, yoga practice has taught me that I have everything inside myself to help me fulfill all the cravings I have in my life.

One of my favorite indicators that yoga gives is my perfectly imperfect body. My friends tell me about their experiences with yoga and how they have had a great time discovering who they are. To encounter this self-knowing feeling in any pose is similar to the feeling of being liberated. I could not imagine anything better than having a model-like physique in the beginning. In the same way, my friends wanted the same. Thankfully, that desire no longer overwhelms us as such desires always end up making you feel uncomfortable and unsatisfied. We have found much more than just a physique through our yoga practice.

Many people show up for their first yoga class thinking that I will assist them in achieving their ideal body shape or, if nothing else, dialing back their growing age marks on their bodies. So, do I help them? Well, I assist them with doing whatever they desire, just not in the manner they want! I try to give them the opportunity to have something more than what they want. I want them to feel the inconspicuous, inward progression of energy that signifies a new world opening inside them.

The essential truth is that there could be nothing "greater" than yoga. The point is to meet yourself in the reality of who you "truly" are with affection, acknowledgment, and comprehension. You look intently in the mirror and see a lot deeper than the skin and more profoundly than the kinks of the different life experiences.

There is a heavenly quality to all bodies. Through yoga, we are usually reminded that we live inside our body and associate it with our embodiment. These feelings are a huge source of calmness, especially growing old.

Yoga is about truth; it is about looking at yourself and saying this to yourself: "This is the sort of person I am, flawed, but still, I am perfect in myself. There is a hallowed quality to all bodies, including my own." Yoga makes you fall in love with yourself, and with age, loving yourself becomes quite difficult (A bitter reality).

You are not intended to create altered forms of yourself ever in your life. Confidence should be an everyday constant even as you age, and respect and empathy for you and others should be fundamental to each day. With yoga, you learn how to open your heart to yourself and others and realize that you are enough for yourself. Moreover, it fends off the diseases from your mind and body and fortifies your body while providing you with a sense of prosperity and strength. Well, you are in a win-win situation with yoga.

Moreover, yoga helps hone our thinking capacity and develop our brains as we grow old. We can accomplish a more significant level of focus through yoga and regulate our feelings much better even after 50. It helps us interact more with nature and upgrades our social prosperity.

Also, you can learn self-control and mindfulness through yoga whenever you practice it consistently. Therefore, you will acquire a positive force inside yourself once you do yoga, which will assist you in having a healthy life liberated from any issues.

Yoga is an incredible gift to humans. It assists us in making our lives better and keeping up with our well-being. One fosters a higher tolerance level when practicing yoga, which helps ward off negative thoughts and get a better understanding of life, which clears their mind.

To put it simply, yoga has many advantages, as discussed in the previous chapter. Everybody should try and practice it daily to maintain their fitness and benefit from it. It is the key to a long and healthy life without the utilization of any unnatural things such as drugs. This chapter will give you more details on the impact of different aspects of yoga movements on your body and the healthy body mechanisms. Hop on to the section below!

2.1 Movement – An Anti-Aging Medicine

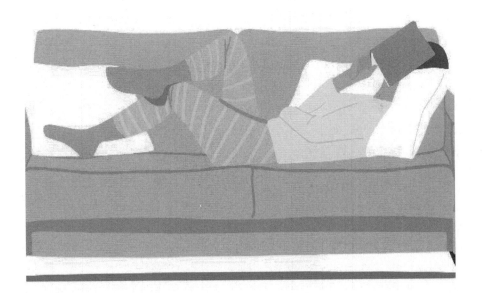

Movement is basic yet extremely important for a healthy life after 50. Our bodies are intended to move in many diverse ways. We run, jump, walk, swim, bend forward or backward, etc. If you are 50 or above and feel lazy working out every day, then you need to read this section carefully and understand the importance of movement. It is an ideal opportunity to quit considering the everyday practice as an enormous and gigantic task such as running five miles on your first day of running. Rather, your practice sessions can and should be undeniably less burdening with little steps in the right direction to accommodate your body's health level.

In the modern routine, an average individual sits for up to 10-13 hours a day, but our ancestors used to work in the fields and would eventually end up resting for only 3-4 hours each day. In addition, they would go everywhere on foot. Unfortunately, we do not have such levels of physical movement which is crucial to maintaining a healthy lifestyle.

Moving is a central part of life and includes much more than just workouts. It does not need heavy exertion and only requires activity. Movement influences everything, from blood flow to cellular processing to digestion to immunity. With movement, our bodies manage chemical reactions, detoxify our bodies and revitalize our muscles and organs. Everyday activity increases synthetic changes in the body and animates neural pathways, which incites our working limit and enhances resistance. Movement is fundamental for learning and increases our cerebral working capacity. When we become sluggish, our health becomes compromised, and we need to keep these points in mind, especially after 50.

Practicing yoga is the best safeguard against physical deterioration due to aging. It cannot reverse aging, yet there is evidence that yoga can develop the conditions and resources vital for DNA to fix different cellular mechanisms. Obviously, the sooner you start practicing the exercises and the more you remain active, the better. However, your age should not hold you back from practicing yoga given its universal benefits for people of every age. Research on the impacts of yoga activity on nursing-home inhabitants in Europe clearly showed enhancements in their physical and intellectual capacities just as in their psychological well-being.

Another thing to remember is that the danger of Alzheimer's sickness, cardiovascular infection, Type 2 diabetes, or different challenges of aging may not significantly develop until middle age or later. Practicing yoga and making it a part of your everyday life can help you effectively delay the signs of aging as lifestyle factors can play a significant role in reducing the probability of diseases in life.

Fortunately, you do not need to run a long distance or go to the recreational center to receive the counter-maturing rewards of movement. All you need to do is perform yoga using your whole body which will give you all the physical and intellectual benefits you need, as long as you do it consistently. The body losses old bone tissue and replaces it with new bone tissue to keep bones strong. However, around the age of 30, the new bone tissues slow down in replacing the old ones. As a result, in your 40s and 50s, you gradually lose more bone mass than you make. Exercise can assist your body in keeping the thickness of your bones intact and yoga poses can help your body fight off Osteoporosis, an infection that debilitates bone and increases the likelihood of bone fractures as you age.

As individuals age, they lose their muscles' size and strength, a condition known as Sarcopenia. Researchers say yoga is probably an ideal way to assist with such a condition as it keeps muscle strength and power, and makes routine activities like cleaning, cooking, and climbing steps less troublesome. It can also assist with lessening weakness from sickness, further develop mental well-being and disposition, and assist one in keeping up with their health for a more extended period.

Since osteoporosis influences women more regularly than men, yoga postures are particularly significant before and after menopause. You will get more detailed exercise poses for menopause in the following chapter. While older individuals cannot replace bone mass at an accelerated rate, active yoga practice can assist in forestalling bone fractures and pains. Yoga, when joined with weight-bearing activities, can further assist with developing equilibrium and stability, lessening the risks of falls and breaks.

Telomeres play a significant role in cell regulations. They are the covers on the ends of DNA strands, like the covers on shoelaces. Their length diminishes with age, and this adds to cell senescence or deterioration. In addition, telomere length is associated with specific ongoing conditions, particularly hypertension, stroke, and coronary illness. A few investigations have discovered that yoga therapies are connected with longer telomere lengths in particular individuals. This is by all accounts particularly obvious in aged individuals.

As researchers keep on exploring the impacts of yoga, they are tracking down a wide range of invigorating advantages. For example, research claims that practicing yoga produces myokines, little proteins with a wide range of advantages to your mind such as improved brain function, positive effect on the nature of your sleep, protection from neuronal injury, and improved learning and locomotive activity.

There is still a ton we do not know about the effects of yoga on the aging system. However, we know this: moving your body consistently five times each week, for thirty minutes every day, is better than moving it on rare occasions. The benefits of practicing yoga are impressive, and it feels like being born again. The best part is that it is never too late to practice yoga!

2.2 Healthy Body Mechanics

The term "body mechanics" refers to the manner in which we move while performing our typical activities, such as sitting, standing, sleeping, and walking. If we utilize poor body mechanics, this can frequently result in back problems. The spine is subjected to abnormal pressures when we move improperly or unsafely, and eventually, this can cause spinal structures such as discs and joints to deteriorate. As a result, learning good body mechanics is critical. Once you become accustomed to them, incorporating them into your daily routine should be relatively easy.

- **Standing**

Many individuals spend a lot of time on their feet. Standing covers bending, lifting, and doing different other works with the help of your feet. It can sometimes be hard on the back, particularly when the proper body mechanics are not utilized. The following rules can be utilized to limit the risk of injury to your back when completing any tasks that require you to stand on your feet.

> - *Try not to remain in one posture for an extended period of time.*
> - *Change your way of standing as frequently as possible. This will not just assist you in easing weight on your spine but also help with lessening muscle weariness.*
> - *Try to stretch whenever you can. Delicate stretching practices throughout a break can assist with easing muscle snugness.*
> - *Take care of the surface you are standing upon. Make sure it is firm and level.*

While lifting an item, abstain from bowing and turning abruptly. Instead, make sure you face the object, move close to it, and bend through your knees into a squat position. Make sure your feet are leveled on the floor and are shoulder-width apart. In a continuous gentle motion, lift up by straightening your knees without a hitch. Utilize a similar technique when putting the objects down.

Abstain from overreaching to pick anything up. If you need to still do it, make sure you are standing on a firm surface. Try not to remain in any unnecessarily stretched position for long as it can put a needless strain on the back and neck.

- **Poses or postures**

We have all been told since adolescence to "stand upright." However, it is very easy to get into the unfortunate quirks. Great body mechanics depend on a great pose or posture. A great posture means that the spine is in an "unbiased" position, i.e., not excessively adjusted forward or curved back. It is simple to maintain a good posture; follow the technique below.

> - *Stand with your feet separated.*
> - *Make a little curve in your lower back by turning the pelvis into a neutral position where it is slightly tilting forwards. Be mindful so as not to curve excessively.*
> - *Lift your chest up and pull the shoulders back.*

This is how you get a good posture! Do you feel how adjusted and leveled your spine is? Practice this posture until it starts to feel natural. Monitoring your pose during every yoga session is an ideal way to ensure you utilize great body mechanics.

- **Sleeping**

We spend around 33% of our day in bed, so we cannot overlook how our bodies are situated when we are sleeping. Similar to waking hours, the objective here is to keep a straight spine while we sleep. This can be done by:

> - *Making sure you are resting on a solid sleeping cushion.*
> - *Avoiding to sleep on your belly or using a high pillow to prop up your head since these positions can result in your*

back being bent and unnecessary pressure being exerted on
your spine.

- *To maintain a neutral spine, it is highly recommended for individuals with back or neck problems to adopt the side or back positions.*

- *Placing a cushion between or behind your knees is an effective way to stabilize your spine and alleviate lower back discomfort.*

- *Opt for a pillow that allows your head to stay aligned with your body for optimal spinal alignment.*

- *Various large cushions might look extraordinary on a made bed, however, they do not benefit your back while sleeping, so try to avoid them where possible.*

- **Sitting**

Regardless of whether one is sitting in the work area or at home watching the TV, it is vital to remember great body mechanics. For deskwork, think about investing in an ergonomic chair and an adjustable desk. What does appropriate sitting resemble?

- *Sitting with your buttocks at the back of the chair, ensuring a slight gap between your knees and the seat.*

- *Keeping your feet flat on the ground with your knees forming a 90-degree angle.*

- *Retracting the shoulders, bringing back the chest.*

If your chair has armrests, make sure they are adjusted to help with the weight of your arms. Not too high that they make you hunch and not too low that you end up slouching. Hassocks can also be used to help keep up with a great stance while sitting.

To prevent strain on your lower back during extended sitting periods, it is important to have adequate support. Consider finding a chair that allows for adjustable lumbar support. If this is not feasible, you can still provide support with a lumbar roll or by placing a rolled-up towel or cushion behind your lower back. However, keep in mind that maintaining the correct sitting position for prolonged periods can be difficult, so it is important to take breaks, move around, and stretch to reduce the strain on your spine and prevent your muscles from becoming fatigued and stiff.

As it may be obvious by now, the correct body mechanics are essential for keeping your body healthy and they are not difficult to incorporate into your daily routine. They might feel or appear unnatural at the start, but if you keep practicing them, they will handily become everyday practice. Trust me, your body will thank you for these adjustments!

2.3 Partnering with Yoga for Life

Partnering with yoga would become the best choice for your life. As mentioned earlier, recent research shows that practicing yoga actively benefits individuals with psychological well-being issues and removes burdensome manifestations in them. In any case, yoga assists with an entire scope of physical and mental well-being issues, particularly after the worldwide well-being emergency.

The COVID pandemic shackled the world, and most of us were shocked. With everything shutting down on us, we required a getaway to life and happiness. So, the majority went to yoga and exercise to get fit and relax their mind from all the world's troubles.

Yoga has been an unshakable decision of life taken by teachers to various specialists since the days of yore. Yoga is not just an enormous type of activity but an ideal strategy to keep your psychological and mind's capacities sound and generous.

In our busy, unpleasant daily schedule, amid the hustle of work, we regularly let things that matter blur into the commotion. Our psyches are continually on the move; however, our bodies are frequently not. We have attempted tedious eating routines and a wide range of fasting. However, all of this has only led to more negatives. The COVID pandemic is practically similar to a reminder to wake us up and make a stride toward a better living technique. Remaining fit does not really mean accomplishing the sculpted physique or having the best pair of abs. Contrary to prevalent thinking, wellness is a blend of our true healthy selves, and it is nothing but the truth that yoga is the ideal fit for our dull and unhealthy lives.

Yoga is not just an impetus in our wellness excursion, but it also helps our brain and inward well-being. Relaxing is an essential piece of yoga. It helps us stay focused and has been demonstrated to further develop our body while reducing any stress. The quietness with which one practices yoga permits the brain to gather its musings and speak with them. It clears up a stage for thought, makes one less receptive to an ominous example, and, in particular, interfaces the individual to their actual self.

As far as we might be concerned, life can become unremarkable with dull schedules and a perishing interest. The compensating practice of yoga and its slow-paced Asanas helps us familiarize the outside self with the complicated inside. Standard reflection permits the brain to move away from the consistent issue and snare of thoughts. It allows the psyche to focus on one idea and questions its material presence.

Yoga helps us reach our spirit by connecting the brain with the body. The act of yoga is a satisfying encounter that just the devoted person can understand. Yoga is not only an activity structure but also a type of lifestyle. Yoga is an elective life structure that would lead individuals to a better way of life and help them heal spiritually.

The sacredness of yoga is the sole variable that connects individuals from varying backgrounds. It has started a trend that no other type of activity at any point could. Yoga is helping out millions in overcoming issues between what the body says and what the brain needs!

Chapter 3: Relaxing into Life with Yoga

Sometimes we all get immensely involved in our hectic life to meet different work and life expectations and pressures. In such situations, we usually forget to relax. However, relaxing for only five minutes occasionally can lower feelings of anxiety and stress, and give us the energy we really need to handle the different challenges we are facing.

Stress is not always terrible for health! A specific measure of pressure is important to manage challenging situations in our daily lives and to become more resilient. Different hormonal and physical changes in our bodies make us feel DIFFERENT. Sometimes this "unusual or different feeling" makes us feel good. Change is important for everyday life, however, if we are always in a state of high stress and anxiety, it can cause a lot of harm to our brains and body. So, knowing and bearing the right amount of stress is very important in life.

Relaxing is a state in which you feel calm, and content, which is quite important, especially if you have a busy routine. It has numerous physical and psychological medical benefits as it helps you deal with any stress or uneasiness in life. Relaxing diminishes the pressure and the side effects of psychological conditions like hopelessness, nervousness, and schizophrenia. Its other medical benefits include:

- *Bringing down your pulse, circulatory strain, and breathing rate*
- *Decreasing muscle strain and constant agony*
- *Developing focus and disposition*

Different relaxing procedures focus on calming the muscles and the systems of the body. Find a method for relaxation that works for you and make it part of your daily schedule, regardless of whether it is only for five to ten minutes every day. Always remember that keeping a healthy balance between serious and fun activities assists your body in reducing stress and relaxing.

Physical issues, such as migraines, strains in the shoulders or neck, dazedness, and exhaustion, are all a consequence of stress and over-burden. Stress can also influence our psychological state as it lifts cortisol levels. This can bring about nervousness, trouble in making decisions, and wild and negative thoughts. Also, to add to the list, other problems can present as irritability, sensations of being overpowered, low confidence, and sorrow. Extreme stress in an individual can lead to aggressive behavior, wrong correspondence, drinking excessive amounts of liquor, smoking, and worsening of disposition.

Being stressed for extended periods can cause tiredness and weakness. As per some psychologists, the results of pressure chemicals can start acting as tranquilizers (synthetic substances which make us mentally exhausted and fall unconscious) in the body. When such chemicals are released in significant quantities, which will occur under states of constant pressure, they can result in a feeling of low energy, weakness, or hopelessness.

We cannot always stay away from pressure; however, figuring out how to handle stress in life is very critical! Relaxing plays a fundamental role in controlling pressure. When we relax, there is an increase in the flow of blood around our brain and body, which gives us more energy. In addition, it assists us with settling our minds which helps in thinking positively and focusing and supports our memory and navigation.

Relaxing eases back our pulse and heart rate, diminishes our circulatory strain, and alleviates cardiovascular pressure. It also helps process food as we absorb nutrients more effectively when relaxed, which also assists with warding off sickness and illness. Therefore, whenever you are in a tricky situation, try to relax even if it is for five minutes. This can diminish the feelings of anxiety and give your energy levels a lift. Here are a few relaxing methods that are fast and simple to do:

- *Focus on your breathing and take deep breaths.*
- *Moderately relax your muscles (tighten and loosen up your muscles all through your body.)*
- *Work on your imagination and try to calm yourself through positive thinking.*
- *Go for a peaceful stroll and appreciate natural beauty.*

Take control of your life by following a relaxation program that fulfills your mental needs because this in itself is very empowering. It is genuinely essential to try and relax at home as well. There are numerous straightforward and economical ways of having a little relaxing time in your life including giving time to music, going for a little walk by yourself in the park, reading a good book, being imaginative, having a little chat with close friends or colleagues, working out, cleaning up, or whatever assists you in relaxing your mind and body.

Relaxing is easy and essential for a healthy brain and body. When we do not talk about relaxing, it usually appears to be something that we are not ready to fit into our timetables. It is perhaps one of the best things to fuse into your daily routine. Constant stress and pressure can negatively affect both your physical and emotional well-being, so, it is important to start relaxing, fellas!

Yoga is one of the most famous relaxing methods around the world. In yoga, different poses can assist with reducing numerous persistent issues in your body. It helps in reestablishing energy levels and empowering self-appreciation so continue reading this chapter that is all about various yoga poses for different illnesses, sicknesses, and problems. Enjoy reading further!

3.1 Yoga for Beginners

If you are new to yoga, it can feel confusing and hard to know precisely where and how to begin. This yoga basics section has been explicitly written for beginners like yourself to give you the tips, rules, and techniques you need to start practicing beneficial yoga poses at home. I recommend reading this whole section before engaging in any of the yoga poses mentioned below to guarantee your prosperity and prevent any injury.

Yoga is a tremendous assortment of profound strategies and practices pointed toward incorporating the mind, body, and soul to accomplish a condition of improvement or unity with the universe. The various ways of yoga accentuate multiple methodologies and strategies that lead to a similar objective of unification and illumination. What has ordinarily been considered yoga in Western countries is the "Hatha" yoga, or the yoga of force, which is one of the numerous ways of yoga.

Hatha yoga achieves the association of brain, body, and soul through an act of Mudra (body motions or gestures), Pranayama (yoga breathing or practice of breathing regulation), Shatkarma (interior purging or cleansing practices), and Asanas. These yoga practices are used to clean the body and develop Prana (life-empowering energy).

If your body is rigid, I suggest you start with delicate and easy practice until you have developed the grit and adaptability for challenging poses or postures. If you are moderately fit and flexible, you should have the option to bounce squarely into a regular Hatha yoga class. I suggest you avoid Bikram, Hot Yoga, or Ashtanga until you have developed some fortitude and perseverance in your body. As a beginner, you should approach yoga gradually and cautiously. The ideal way to know which yoga is for you is to check the basic poses!

Yoga is ordinarily done with bare feet on a tacky yoga mat with discretionary yoga props, and garments that can stretch easily with your body. You can easily assemble a stretchable outfit from your closet to get everything rolling or buy clothing that is explicitly intended for yoga practice from any nearby shopping store. Yoga classes might use a few extra props with the most well-known being square boxes, covers, and blocks. You do not have to buy these immediately as you can undoubtedly substitute these things with scarves or ties, a heap of books, and cushions.

I suggest starting with a short and direct yoga practice and gradually developing from that point. When you feel comfortable with a couple of essential beginner yoga postures, you can fuse them into succession and keep on adding additional challenging poses. Make sure you learn and follow the fundamental parts of yoga, including breathing, reflection, expectation, and relaxation. Following are some basic yoga poses that you can start with.

1. Mountain Pose (Tadasana)

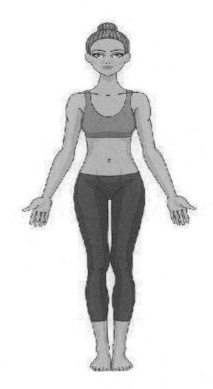

Assume a stance with your feet together on the mat. Lower your shoulder blades towards your back, and keep your shoulders away from your ears. Gently elevate the top of your head. Join your thighs, contract your tummy, and ease your arms to your sides with palms directed forward while lengthening your spine. Unclench your jaw and smoothen your forehead. Then, arch your chest upwards while taking slow breaths.

It might appear as though you are simply floating. Just calm your mind. This basic pose will help you increase flexibility in your body. It advances balance and guides your focus toward the good things in life.

2. Downward Facing Dog (Adho Mukha Svanasana)

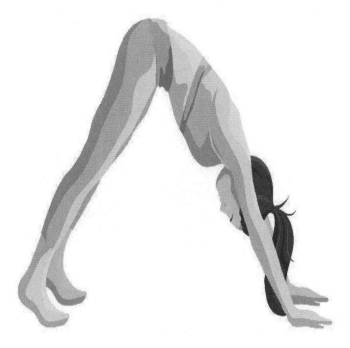

Bend forward at your back to touch the ground. Lay down if necessary. Fold your toes and lift your hips up and back to extend your spine. If your hamstrings are tight, keep your knees bent to bring your weight once more into the legs. Spread your fingers wide, press into the floor with your hands, and pivot your arms with the aim that the biceps are pointing toward each other. Stretch your thighs behind you.

This pose is called the bread and butter of yoga which opens your shoulders, protracts your spine, and stretches your hamstrings. Since your head is underneath your heart, the gentle reversal makes a relaxing impact.

3. Chair Pose (Utkatasana)

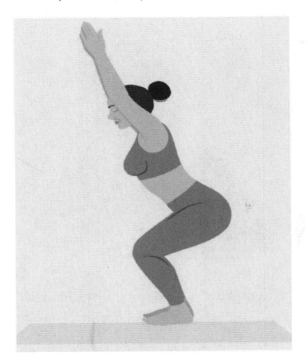

Begin by practicing the mountain pose, wherein you inhale, elevate your arms, unfurl your fingers, and extend upward through your fingertips. Upon exhaling, briefly pause and descend as if settling into a chair. Proceed to shift your weight towards your heels and extend your spine upwards. Inhale and raise your arms while extending them, and exhale while delving deeper into the posture. This invigorating stance will strengthen your legs, upper back, and shoulders, and offer an opportunity to enhance your pliability as your thighs relax. It's important to remain relaxed throughout the process.

4. Hero Pose (Virasana)

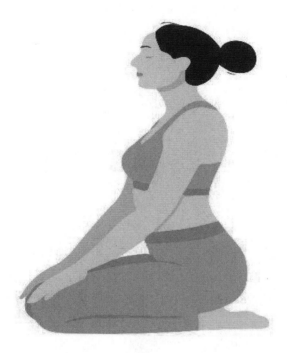

Sit on the yoga mat in a kneeling position with your knees together and your feet directly under you or on your sides. As you breathe out, sit deeper into the position so you feel a nice stretch. Remain in this pose for one minute or more and continue to breathe. As you get comfortable with this position, try spreading your feet apart so you can sit deeper in the space between your feet. Make sure that your feet are pointing straight back and not turning outward or inward.

A posture with "hero" in its name may not sound very harmonious, yet this sitting posture can help quiet thoughts and calm your mind while fortifying your legs and improving your body's endurance.

5. Down Dog on a Seat (Adho Mukha Svanasana)

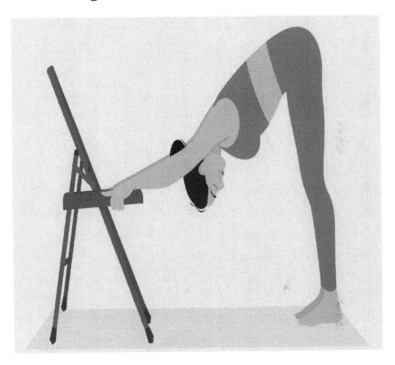

It is a variation of the normal downward-facing dog. Kneel in front of a chair and place your hands on the chair shoulder distance apart. Gradually slide back with your knees as you hinge at your hips until you make a right angle between your thighs and belly such that your spine is parallel with the floor. Lift through your thighs and stand on your feet. Tuck your arms in and extend through your belly, lifting your belly button up towards the ceiling. Relax for a few seconds and then slowly lower down to the starting position.

Remember that yoga is highly beneficial. Regardless of what people say about it, I advise you that yoga asana is not about flawlessness. It is all about progress. It is tied in with making peace with the awkwardness that comes when you start performing yoga. It is about an association with the brain and body, mainly protecting your body. Whether you start performing yoga on a mat and lie in Savasana (corpse pose) for 15 minutes, or indulge in some of the more complex poses, you are still doing yoga, fellas.

3.2 Yoga for Meditation

After coming home from work, there is a time when your life feels like a non-stop highway of events. Life is continuous, and at times you simply need a second to treat yourself. This is the time when yoga proves to be extremely useful, and I am here to teach you some of the best yoga poses for meditation that can enable you to relax after a long busy day.

Stress is not only in your mind but it can also influence your body. It can cause strain, particularly in your neck, face, and lower and upper back. So, before you can clear your mind with yoga, you will have to bring your body into a condition of serenity and relinquish it. Following are two main types of meditation practices.

1. Concentration Meditation

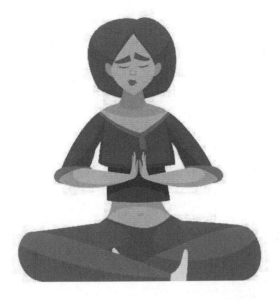

This type of medication includes concentrating on a focal point. This could involve following the breathing rhythm, continuously repeating a mantra or any word, gazing at a light fire, paying attention to a monotonous gong, or counting dabs on a chain. Since keeping your brain concentrating on a single thing is quite testing, a person who has just started practicing this meditation may only be able to focus for a couple of moments, but with regular practice, they can concentrate for longer periods.

In this meditation practice, you bring back your mind to the selected object of consideration each time you notice your brain is meandering and instead of focusing on irregular contemplations or thoughts, you essentially let them go. Through this cycle, you will be able to considerably improve your capacity to focus.

2. Mindful Meditation

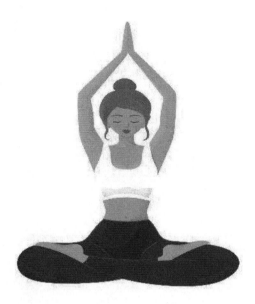

The practice of this meditation encourages individuals to observe their wandering thoughts and ideas without getting entangled in them or making any judgments. Instead, they are advised to acknowledge each psychological note as it arises. By doing so, one can gain an understanding of how their thoughts and feelings tend to fluctuate. Over the long haul, you can become more mindful of human habits such as rapid passing of judgment on an encounter as fortunate or unfortunate or charming or not. Moreover, by practicing this type of meditation every day, you can form an internal equilibrium inside your brain that can help you be calmer and more composed.

In certain schools, many students practice a blend of concentration meditation and mindful meditation. These meditation types can have many different procedures and practices. For instance, the everyday practice of meditation among Buddhist priests centers around the development of empathy. This includes imagining adverse occasions and reevaluating them in a positive light by changing them through empathy.

Many scientists are presently investigating whether a steady meditation practice yields long-term benefits and are noticing beneficial outcomes on the mind such as a higher resilience and thinking capacity among meditators. However, the motivation behind most meditation is not to accomplish such benefits, rather it is essentially done just to be present in the moment.

A definitive advantage of meditation is the brain's freedom from connection to things it cannot handle, like strong inner or outer feelings. As a result, people who practice yoga do not unnecessarily follow or stick to certain negative encounters. Instead, they keep a quiet brain and emotion of concordance, bringing true strength to their body. Since you now have all the information regarding meditation, it is an ideal opportunity to kick some unnecessary stuff out of your mind with some of the best meditation yoga poses.

- **Full Lotus Pose (Padmasana)**

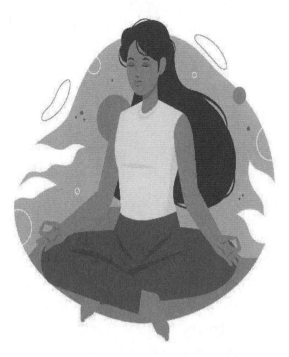

This pose is a traditional pose for meditation yoga and requires adaptability, focus, and commitment to perform it perfectly. Take a seated position on a mat with legs extended forward. Proceed to bend your right knee and place your right foot upon your left thigh. Subsequently, bend your left knee and place your left foot on your right thigh. Draw in a full breath and unite your body in calmness while performing the pose. Focus your brain on breathing and think about what you might want to accomplish after meditation. This is a powerful posture, so you may only be able to hold it for a brief moment. Try switching your legs from the left one up to the right one so you can extend your meditation.

- **Burmese Position (Sukhasana)**

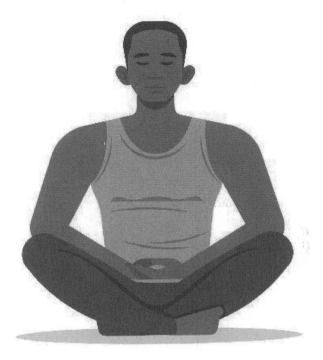

This position allows your body to calm down to utilize the entire focus at the forefront of your thoughts. To get in this position, take place on your mat. Your legs should be crossed, and your feet should be tenderly intersected in the center. Next, place your hands softly on your thighs, and take a full breath such that it tops your body off with oxygen; then, slowly exhale. Keep repeating this cycle again and again while keeping your mind concentrated on your objectives.

- **Seiza Position (Vajrasana)**

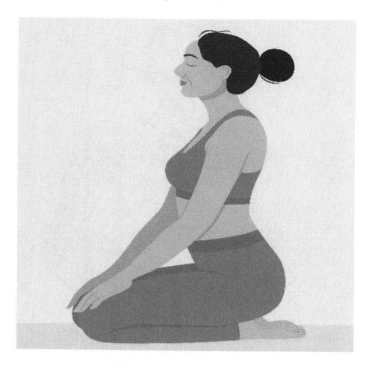

Seiza is a traditional way of sitting in which one kneels to keep their back straight and their mind clear. Start with kneeling on the mat with both of your feet tucked under your bum; for additional support, a pad can be put in the space between your bum and legs. Keep your back straight, shut your eyes, put your hands on your lap, and take full breaths. Make sure you clear your mind and concentrate just on a single thought.

Meditation might offer a solution for the growing need to alleviate pressure amidst occupied timetables and busy lives by focusing and connecting with our thoughts. Meditation poses require various abilities and attitudes, and similar to yoga, it is not intended to be something forceful or strenuous. If it feels forced, it will turn into a duty, and one would not be able to practice it regularly. So, it is important to recognize when mediation is becoming difficult and challenging and be prepared to take breaks as needed. This will turn an ordinary meditation practice into a beautiful and enjoyable time. There are countless types of meditation, so if one is not working or is not satisfying your needs, you can simply go for a different one.

3.3 Yoga for Devotion

Devotional yoga is one of the fundamental yogic ways that leads to enlightenment. This kind of yoga signifies "dedication" or "love". Bhakti, devotional worship which is directed to a deity, is viewed as the simplest yogic way to unite the body, soul, and mind. Unlike other types of yoga that require a solid and adaptable body or a trained and robust mind, Bhakti yoga requires an open and adoring heart.

This beautiful yoga practice focuses vigorously on the Hindu pantheon of deities. Every one of these deities is viewed as addressing a delicate part of the single divine figure (God) or Brahman similar to how the Christians address explicit traits and characteristics of God. It must be noted here that for devotional yoga, it is not necessary to use one of the Hindu deities. One just needs to find their object of devotion, which can be even more compelling in achieving the benefits of this type of yoga.

There are nine principal practices of Bhakti yoga that can be practiced either independently or combined. Each of these practices makes a particular Bhava, a mindful intent or emotion that creates a mental space or a mood for yoga, that can enable yogis to elevate their relationship with the object of their devotion. Following are nine different practices of devotional yoga:

1. **Padasevana** – *These practices consolidate the act of bhakti (dedication) with karma yoga (benevolent help). The yogi expresses their love for the deity or the object of their devotion through service such as volunteering, helping someone in need, or simply spreading love.*

2. **Vandana** – *this is one's "surrender" before the divine in the form of a prayer to limit self-centeredness and self-absorption.*

3. **Shravana** - *This practice includes listening to sacred writings including stories and poems by a saint (Bhakta) in a group with other devotees.*

4. **Smarana** - *In this practice, the divine is remembered and kept at the forefront of one's mind by continually reflecting upon the diety's name and characteristics.*

5. **Archana** - *This practice involves worshiping the object of devotion to purify the heart through love and respect.*

6. **Atmanivedana** - *This practice includes complete surrender of oneself to the Divine or object of devotion.*

7. **Dasya** – *Focuses on the unquestioning dedication to the divine, including serving the desire of God rather than one's inner desire.*

8. **Kirtana** - *This practice focuses on devotional songs and praises that are typically rehearsed in an "action and reaction" manner with the yogi singing or chanting in response to another chant or praise.*

> 9. **Sakhya** - *This practice includes the fellowship and relationship between the Divine and the yogi.*

The most famous practice of Bhakti Yoga in the West is Kirtana (typically called Kirtan), in which mantras are chanted using classical Indian musical instruments. Kritan can be practiced without help from anyone and can be coordinated into different yoga practices. The advantages of devotional yoga are enormous. It relaxes the heart and eliminates envy, contempt, desire, outrage, selfishness, pride, and egotism. It implants satisfaction, divine joy, ecstasy, harmony, and love in the hearts of those individuals that practice this yoga every day. All considerations, stresses and tensions, fears, mental tortures, and afflictions disappear entirely with the help of this yoga.

3.4 Yoga for Better Posture

Many believe that sitting continuously for hours is the new smoking (fashionable yet very unhealthy). Sitting continuously for extended periods and having a sedentary lifestyle can adversely affect an individual's health that goes beyond one's eyes. It also negatively influences digestion and posture, increases nervousness and sadness, and can also prompt weight gain. Terrible postures can prompt complex issues like back pain, cardiovascular problems, and digestion issues. In the long run, poor postures can change the shape of the spine which can result in permanent, long-term back issues. Studies have shown that a bad posture can also change the way others see you and can make you appear less enthusiastic or older than your age.

Yoga can be a great method for combatting the adverse consequences of sitting in a work area in a bad posture for a long period of time. For example, heart-opener yoga poses, often used to describe chest-opening or back-bending postures, are known to fix various issues related to a bad posture problem while also providing emotional and spiritual healing.

There are eight types of yoga poses you can practice to fix bad postures. These yoga poses can be practiced one at a time or can be combined together based on what feels best for one's body and helps the most in fixing bad posture problems. Practice the following yoga positions routinely during breaks from work or whenever you want a decent stretch in your body!

1. Cow Face Arms (Gomukhasana)

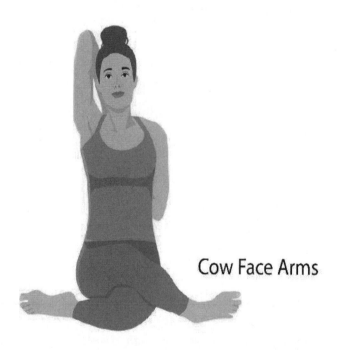

Cow Face Arms

This pose can be practiced at any time, even at work, and works phenomenally when you are sat on your lounge chair. While sitting on a chair, lift your right arm up and bend it towards the back as if you are trying to scratch down your back. Next, sweep your left arm up your back and try to grab your right hand with your left. If you cannot get your hands to touch, just hold a rope or a cloth between your hands and repeat the process while slowly trying to reduce the gap between your hands. Next, lift your chest up and try to relax in this position for five deep breaths, and then let go. To make the pose harder, try bending your right knee to cross your right foot over the left leg, with your left foot hanging outside of the right hip. Repeat this as many times as you can, and I am sure you will feel better!

2. Camel Pose (Ustrasana)

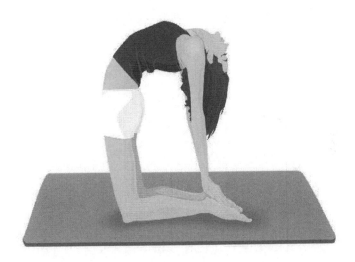

This back bend pose can help with releasing the back after sitting in front of a PC or workstation all day. It opens your heart (chest), shoulders, and throat. There are numerous ways to do this pose. The best variation starts with kneeling on your knees, with toes tucked under your legs.

Next, lifts yourself up by pressing your hips forward and lifting your chest, while ensuring that the shoulders are relaxed and far from the ears. Bend backward to try to touch your feet while pushing your chest up toward the ceiling. Take a deep breath and hold it in for three seconds, then, gradually just breathe out. Repeat the process as many times as needed, and you will feel your pain go away.

3. Heart Bench Pose

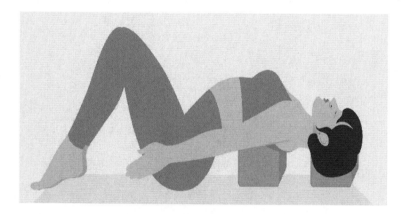

This pose is also known as the supported fish pose, and makes your posture feel astonishing, particularly before bed or after a long vehicle ride. For this posture, you will require two yoga blocks. Set the two blocks on a flat surface in the form of a "T." The long piece of the "T" will rest between your shoulder bones, and the top block (the highest point of the "T") will hold your head. Lay back on the block as you open and stretch your chest, however, make sure that there is no uneasiness, and just find the 'perfect balance.' Loosen up your whole body and pull your shoulders back and away from your ears as you rest your palms down on the flat surface. Take five to ten deep breaths and let go.

4. Cobra Pose (Bhujangasana)

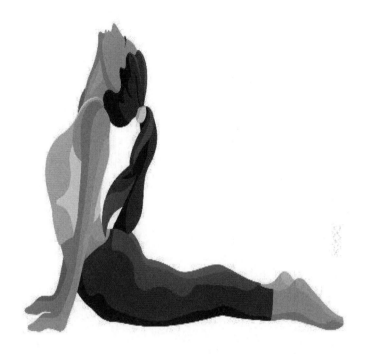

This pose reinforces the arms while opening the upper back and shoulders. Lay back on your belly, your face lying on the ground, the front of your feet level with the floor and place your hands underneath the shoulders. Keep your legs together and allow your feet to touch one another. Spread the fingers wide and push down equally to lift the head, neck, and chest off the mat, keeping your elbows near your body. Press the elbows close to the body's sides and close the jaw without putting much strain on the neck. Keep your shoulders and upper body loose even if it means slightly bending your elbows when you first start practicing this pose. Don't worry, soon you would not have to! Hold for three to five breaths and as you breathe out, gently bring your midsection, chest, and head back to the floor. You will love the results of this pose.

5. Plank Pose (Phalakasana)

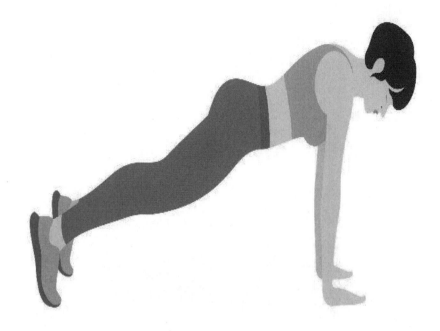

While the Plank pose is not a heart opener, it develops strength, which is a significant part of a healthy posture that will help you stand tall. The most effective method to practice this pose is to lay down on your belly, put the palms of your hands next to your shoulders and spread your fingers wide with your feet shoulder distance apart. Press the floor away with the hands and tighten all muscles in the legs as you lift yourself up from the floor. Once your chest is off the ground, lift your hips up and hold this position while resisting dropping back towards the mat. Hold this pose for thirty seconds, and then let go. Repeat as much as you can!

6. Span Pose (Setu Bandha Savargasasana)

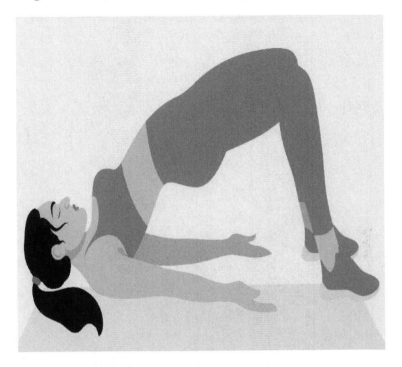

This pose fortifies the lower body while opening the spine and neck, and is an extraordinary backbend for all levels since you can pick how deep to go based on how you feel. Start off by laying on your back, palms facing down at the sides, and feet flat on the floor a little away from the hips. Breathe in, push your hands against the floor to lift your hips up towards the ceiling, and hold this position for three breaths before letting go. Repeat as much as you can.

7. Bow Pose (Dhanurasana)

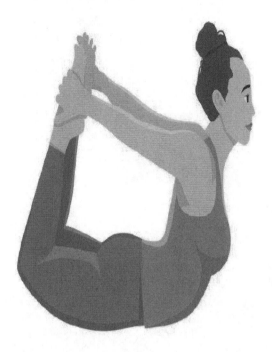

This pose, when practiced appropriately, feels astonishing on your back and chest. Laying on your belly, bring your palms near to your sides with the face laying tenderly on the mat. Bend your knees, drawing the feet towards your bum. Reach back to grab your lower legs, making sure that the knees are as close to each other as possible. Roll your shoulders from the ears towards your back and lift your chest and thighs off the mat at the same time. Take a deep breath in this position and then let go. Practice it again and again until you master the pose.

8. Downward Facing Dog (Adho Mukha Svanasana)

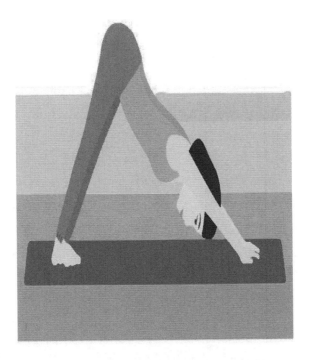

As discussed in section 3.1 of this book, this pose is one of the primary poses we learn in yoga that fortifies the arms, shoulders, and chest and opens up the hamstrings, back, chest, and shoulders. By incorporating it into your daily yoga routine, you can significantly improve your posture.

Yoga is a great way to help reverse the bad posture issue. By fortifying and extending the shoulders, chest, back, and abs (the regions impacted by sitting the entire day), these yoga poses will assist you in standing taller and free from any issues associated with sitting all day. I am sure you will feel relieved after practicing these amazing poses for good postures. So, start practicing today and become healthier!

3.5 Yoga for Bone Diseases

Osteoporosis is a disease where bones become less thick, making them more likely to crack and fracture. Unfortunately, most of the symptoms of osteoporosis are "silent" and usually, individuals are uninformed about this illness unless they specifically run a test for it or have frequent bone breaks. Actively doing exercises is a significant part of the treatment plan for individuals with osteoporosis in which yoga can play an important role. However, just like any exercise, yoga too can result in damage to bones, especially for people suffering from osteoporosis. Therefore, check with your health practitioner to ensure that the yoga is safe for you according to your health to continue your workout. In serious osteoporosis cases, yoga cannot be performed.

Yoga can be advantageous for individuals with early osteoporosis. A report in 2009 confirmed that practicing some yoga poses can build bone thickness when done regularly and appropriately. Some yoga poses further develop stability, equilibrium, and flexibility, which can reduce and even prevent falls, thus reducing and preventing the breakage of bones. Following are some tips you should keep in mind before starting your yoga poses for bone issues and illnesses.

1. *Start slowly and gradually increase the duration of poses as you develop strength, fortitude, and flexibility.*

2. *Continuously practice poses that develop balance to prevent falls and bone breakage, for example, the tree pose, to see long-term benefits and use a block for help if necessary.*

3. Take part in the psychological quietness that comes with yoga if your medical practitioner considers some of the yoga poses to be too risky for you.

4. Incorporate poses that strengthen your hands and arms so they can bear your weight.

5. Focus on poses that develop leg strength, for example, mountain pose, seat posture, and Warrior II.

6. Practice poses that reinforce your back, including some delicate back-bending movements.

7. Continuously keep your spine in a neutral position when practicing different poses.

> **What would be a good idea for you to stay away from?**

1. Sit-ups and crunches as they place a lot of weight on the spine and should be avoided.

2. General poses that require spinal flexion. This implies poses that put unnecessary pressure on the back and can cause it to break.

3. Full backbends.

4. Numerous reversals.

5. Exaggerated turns.

6. Poses that place all of the weight on the hands, like a handstand, as they can put you at an increased risk of a wrist break.

Similar to eating calcium-rich food sources, yoga can be an extraordinary method for alleviating the symptoms and risks of osteoporosis, since numerous yoga poses are known to reinforce the bones and joints as well as calm down an upset mind. The region of the body that are generally impacted the most by bone issues are the spine, wrists, and hips, which can also influence the posture potentially leading to contortions in the body structure. As a result, most yoga has been designed to reinforce the body, particularly in these regions. The following are two yoga poses that will assist with fortifying your bones and building a healthy posture and body structure.

- **Triangle Pose (Trikonasana)**

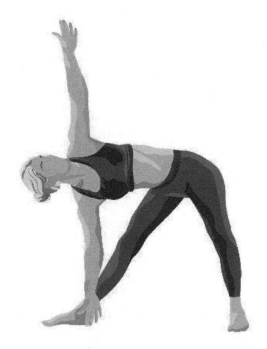

Take a firm and straight standing position with your feet apart, ranging from three and a half to four feet. Rotate your right foot at a 90-degree angle towards your right side and your left foot at a 15-degree angle in the same direction, ensuring that your weight is distributed evenly across both feet. Inhale and exhale deeply as you turn your body to one side, bending at the hips to lower your torso, while keeping your abdomen straight. Stretch your right hand towards the ground and place it outside your right foot or shin, based on your comfort level. Reach upward with your left arm and hold the position, tilting your body sideways instead of forward or backward. As you breathe in and out, gradually get up, bring down your arms, and bring your feet closer. Repeat the process on the opposite side.

- **Chair Pose (Utkatasana)**

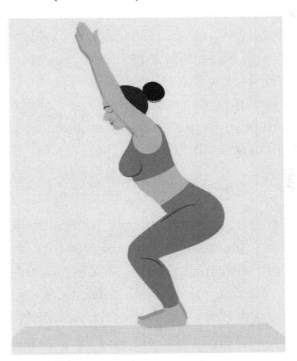

As covered in section 3.1 of this book, stand straight with your feet separated. With your palms facing towards the floor, lift your arms to the front without bending your elbows, until they are parallel to the floor. Gradually bend your knees and lower your pelvis tenderly as though sitting in a chair. To improve the feel of the posture, envision yourself reading a paper or composing on a PC as you stay situated. Make sure your hip does not go past your knees and keep your back and spine straight. Hold this position for a few moments and then slowly rise up.

Yoga can be performed by nearly everybody, as it is very stress-less on the body. However, you might have to practice some easy yoga poses first until you become more comfortable if you experience the ill effects of back pain, and diseases like diabetes retinopathy, or are pregnant (a few asanas may not be permitted for this situation). Therefore, before you start yoga, speak to your primary care physician to understand what you can and cannot do, so you can slowly build your yoga routine which is specific to your needs. While I am sure that yoga will greatly help you, do not use it as a substitute for any medical treatment you are undergoing, rather, use it in addition to your medical treatment to enhance your recovery.

3.6 Yoga for Headaches

Headaches are among the ten leading medical issues in Europe and are possibly the most common reasons for a check-up in general practice and neurological facilities, with as many as around 50% of us experiencing it at least once within the 12 months. These can affect any part of the head or the neck, and therefore, if you experience the ill effects of any standard cerebral pains, you must proceed to look for clinical counsel to learn the type of headache you are experiencing.

Yoga can be an effective tool for the treatment of underlying causes of headaches. Before you can use yoga to treat these issues, you first need to find out why you have severe headaches by looking deeply into your lifestyle. These issues can be caused by extreme stress or tension, and therefore, you need to remove the reason behind your anxiety or stress, which can be done with the help of yoga as it can effectively change the lifestyle of a person. When you start practicing yoga regularly, you will start to feel a visible improvement in your symptoms as your stress fades away and your mental calmness enhances. To improve the effectiveness of yoga for your symptoms, try doing the following before your yoga practice:

1. *Apply some lavender balm as it can help you relax.*

2. *Listen to music that relaxes your mind.*

3. *Get a relaxing neck, shoulder, and head rub.*

Once you feel fully relaxed, try one of the yoga poses detailed below that have been proven to help with headaches.

- **Saga Pose III (Marichyasana III)**

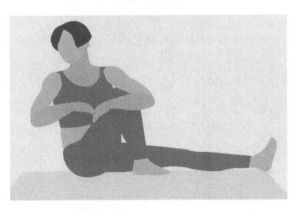

To execute this yoga posture, place your yoga mat near a wall and take a seat, with your legs lying flat on the mat straight in front of you and your back against the wall. Bend your right knee to bring your right foot towards your right hip. Elongate your spine while inhaling and press your palms into the ground. Twist from your pelvis to turn your torso towards the wall and place your left elbow on the outside of your right knee. Open your chest by squaring your shoulder blades with your back ribs. Hold this position for a few breaths. To conclude, release your arm and straighten your leg. Repeat this procedure on the opposite side for a few turns.

- **Butterfly Pose (Baddha Konasana)**

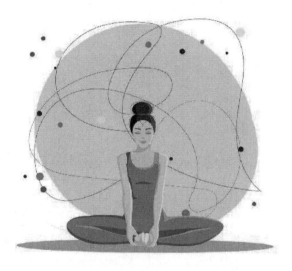

Sit comfortably on a mat and bring your feet together in front of your pelvis to touch your soles, and let your knees drop out to the sides. Fold forward at your hips and let your spine curve as you bring your head close to the floor. Lay down in a forward position from the hips, keeping your spine relaxed and your shoulders wide. Remain in this position for five to ten minutes. Take deep breaths. To release yourself from the position, sit upright, lift your knees to bring your legs into a relaxed position, and then slowly stand up.

- **Forward Bend Pose (Uttanasana)**

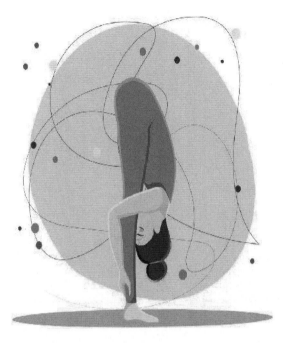

Stand on a mat and take a few deep breaths to relax. As you breathe out, bend forward at your hip to try to touch the floor with your hands. Ensure a gentle bend in your knee joints and maintain a relaxed and ergonomically aligned posture for your spine. If it feels comfortable for you, grab the back of your legs and draw your chest nearer to your shins. Keep your hips over your heels as you press your heels into the floor. Allow your head to hang and keep the neck loose. Extend your spine as you breathe. Hold this position for a few moments before slowly rising back up.

- **Half Lord of Fishes Pose (Ardha Matsyendrasana)**

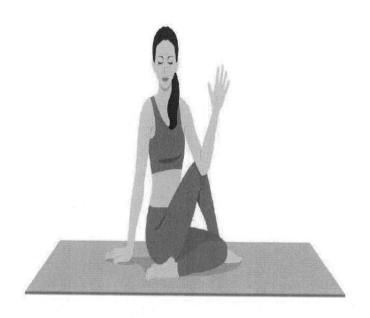

Assume a seated posture on a mat, extending your legs forward. Proceed to raise your right leg and position your right foot to the outside of your left knee. Then, bend your left leg and draw the left foot beneath the right leg to position it outside of the right hip. Inhale deeply, pushing down with your pelvic bone to elongate your spine. Move your right arm to the back of your body and extend your left arm, resting your left elbow upon your right knee. While breathing, twist your torso towards the right, stretching your spine. Stay in this stance for approximately five to eight profound breaths before returning to a neutral position by rotating back to face the center and straightening your legs out in front. Repeat this sequence on the opposite side.

- **Seated Forward Bend Pose (Paschimottonasana)**

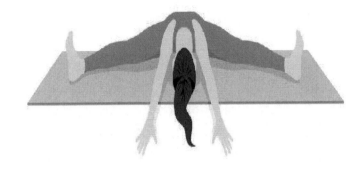

Sit comfortably on a mat with your legs lying flat in front of you. Relax your spine as you breathe, and bend forward, pivoting from the hips as you breathe to grab your toes while keeping a straight back. Allow your arms to relax freely on the floor. If you can touch your feet, great, grab them and slowly pull yourself close to the floor. If you cannot hold your feet, circle a rope around the bottoms of the feet, hold the rope with your hands, and keep your arms straight. With each breath you take in, make sure you stretch out your chest and back and relax. Gradually, move up the rope, closer to your feet so eventually, you can get rid of it. To make this posture even harder, try it with your legs on your side rather than in front of you!

The main element in practicing yoga for headaches is concentrating on breathing. Always remember that if you feel too much pain or discomfort, do not challenge yourself! Instead, gradually improve your flexibility so you can master these poses. The above yoga poses will definitely assist you in alleviating your different issues and symptoms. Simply try these poses and see what works best for you.

3.7 Yoga for Menopause or Andropause

Menopause is when, due to low hormonal levels, periods stop for more than a year. It is preceded by perimenopause, a temporary stage before menopause that has the symptoms of menopause before the periods have actually stopped, which can begin as soon as the age of forty. Perimenopause can have attributes like the start of adolescence where your body goes through a tremendous change including evolving bodies, changing mindsets, and even pimples; however, like everything else, this phase does too pass eventually.

There is an astounding amount of research on menopause available on the internet. You can figure out how to manage symptoms like hot blazes, night sweats, sleeping disorders, weight gain, and vaginal dryness, but, one thing you cannot find is how to "feel" less menopausal. Yoga is a beacon of hope for many transitioning to menopause as yoga for menopause is tied to remaining calm, relaxed, and gathered. It helps you adjust your sensory system and maintain strength without overheating your body. So, start practicing the accompanying four yoga poses that are known to be some of the best ways of managing the symptoms of menopause.

- **Lunge Pose (Banarasana)**

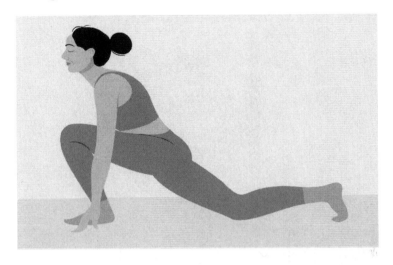

This posture extends and stretches the psoas muscles, which connect the lower back to upper thighs, and hip flexors. The psoas muscles can get tight if one spends most of their day seated with little movement and activity throughout the day. It can also get tight when an individual feels stressed or under pressure. Menopause and its evolving changes can put an individual under a lot of stress which can also lead to shallow breathing. To fix some of these symptoms, it is important to stretch the psoas as they can relax your breath and reduce stress levels, for which, a lunge pose is a great option.

Start on all fours. Lift your right foot and place it in the middle of your hands, making sure that your right knee is directly above the right ankle. Next, start moving your left foot until your left knee is touching the floor and the front of your left foot is lying flat on the floor. Bring your midsection into an upright position with your back straight, and place your hands on your hips. Keep your shoulders loose and look straight ahead. Take a few deep breaths and then repeat on the other side.

- **Forward-Facing Hero Pose (Adho Mukha Virasana)**

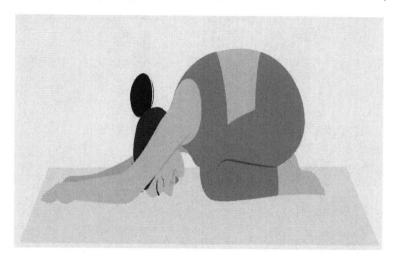

This is outright one of the most loved yoga poses for menopause. It stretches the inner thighs and the spine, stimulates the quad muscles (front of the thighs), and, since the head is lower than the heart, relaxes and cools the sensory system. This pose is great at revitalizing the pelvic area, but make sure to place a rolled-up cover behind your knees if you have knee issues or your thighs are tight.

Start in a kneeling position with your feet touching each other and your torso in an upright position. Bend forwards at your hips, down toward the floor, keeping your spine straight. Stretch your arms forward until you feel a deep stretch in your spine, and place your forehead on the floor between your arms. Relax in this position and take deep breaths.

- **Cow and Cat Pose (Bitilasana Marjaryasana)**

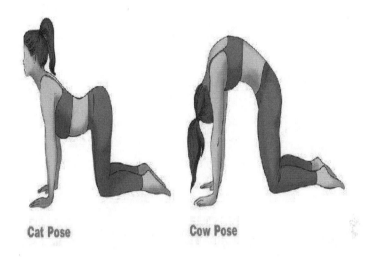

Cat Pose   Cow Pose

These poses move your spine through its full range of movement, extending and stretching both the back and front of your spine. When you broaden your chest in the cat position, you stretch the body parts that are connected with your sympathetic nervous system. This system is a network of nerves that controls your "fight-or-flight" response and is more activated when you are in an emergency, stressed, or in physical danger. As you round your back in a cow pose, you activate the parts of the body that are linked with the parasympathetic sensory system, which controls the opposite response to the sympathetic nervous system which is your calm, relaxed, and quiet reaction. When an individual goes through menopause, their joints begin to dry out which can put an unwanted strain on their nervous system therefore it is important to keep these healthy. This can be achieved by smoothly moving between these two positions, which massage the tissues and joints around the spine while keeping your nervous system healthy, relaxed, and fit.

Start on all fours with your hands directly under your shoulders and your shins gently resting on the floor, with your back straight and your spine in a neutral position. When you start breathing in, curve your back upwards, trying to raise it towards the ceiling, and keep your abs tight. Let your head fall between your arms and lower your gaze. When you start breathing out, drop your spine towards the floor to curve it downwards and raise your head to look forward. Keep your abs and core relaxed while you feel a deep stretch in your back. Repeat these poses a few times and try to coordinate your breathing with your pose change from one to the other.

- **Sphinx Pose (Salamba Bhujangasana)**

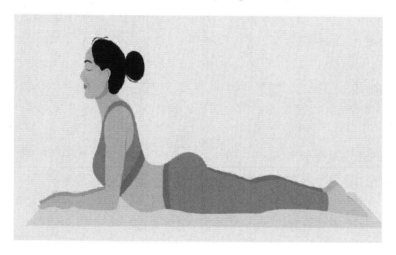

Poses that open the chest up can be a great option to counteract and nullify depression and sluggishness in the body while also stimulating the sympathetic sensory system. These poses, such as the Sphinx pose, are both stimulating and reviving, and energize the individuals who perform them regularly. What makes Sphinx pose so much more useful is that it is a simpler option in contrast to some of the more challenging backbends.

Lying back on your tummy, rest your legs behind you with your front thighs on the floor and feet slightly separated from each other. Lift yourself up by pressing your elbows into the floor, keeping them shoulder distance apart, and fingers spread wide. Try to keep your neck straight as you look forward and feel a deep stretch in your spine. Hold this position for a few moments while breathing deeply and then let go.

Yoga has demonstrated its ability to quieten down the thought process which can give you a minor sensation of uneasiness but will definitely prepare you to deal with your life in a better way. So, give yourself some love and self-care on your yoga mat and feel the benefits that are enjoyed by many. Know about what exacerbates you and what helps you to have an improved outlook, but pay attention and listen to the needs of your body, be alert, and become a successful yogi!

3.8 Yoga for Lung Disease

Yoga is a magnificent type of activity for anybody with Coronary Obstructive Pulmonary Disease (COPD) such as emphysema, long-term bronchitis, and other lung infections. It is low-sway and can assist with working on your physical and emotional well-being. Some of the known benefits of yoga include:

- *Increased levels of relaxation*
- *Reduced pulse or heart rate*
- *Decreased pressure, anxiety, and nervousness*
- *Improved energy levels through enhanced respiration*

Yoga is a mind and body practice. Although its foundations lie in Eastern thinking, anyone can easily start practicing yoga to remain fit, adaptable, flexible, and relaxed. Many yoga poses are available for individuals with medical issues and most of the classes do not focus on the tougher or more strenuous forms of yoga. If you believe you would benefit more from the strenuous yoga poses, feel free to practice them but what is more important is to figure out the type of yoga that works for you.

As discussed in previous chapters, yoga practice is comprised of two fundamental parts: physical stances or poses, known as Asanas, and breathing strategies, known as Pranayamas. Thoughtfulness and relaxation as two additional key pieces which are required for any yoga practice. Practice the following yoga poses to fortify your chest muscles and work on the overall well-being and working of your lungs.

- **Fish Pose (Matsyasana)**

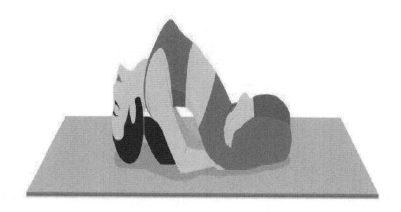

This pose supports deep breathing by extending and reinforcing the lung muscles. It upholds the body's equilibrium, increases oxygen intake, and helps the circulation of blood through the body.

Start with a seated position with your left foot on your right thigh and your right foot on your left thigh. While holding your legs in this crossed position, lie backward on the mat and keep your arms under your body. Lift your chest up, rest your head on the ground while curving your back, and maintain the stability of your entire body using your elbows. Breathe in and breathe out, profoundly opening up the chest. Keep up with this situation however long you are comfortable.

- **Lotus Shoulder Stand Pose (Padma Sarvangasana)**

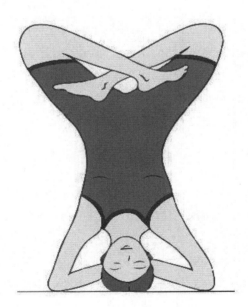

This posture strengthens your diaphragm which improves your breathing over time. Since you are in an upside-down position, there is more pressure on your diaphragm, which pushes into your lungs, and you have to breathe harder to maintain a sufficient level of movement of the air in the lungs. Due to the extra pressure, your intercostal muscles become stronger and your lungs become more efficient. It also helps you develop balance and reinforces the conceptive and sensory systems.

Start with an upheld headstand. If it is too difficult, start by leaning against a wall and use cushions or rolled-up blankets to support you. When you inhale, bend your legs and cross them to bring your left lower leg onto the right thigh and your right lower leg onto the left. Support your back with your hands, and stand firm in this position for a couple of deep breaths or as long as you can hold and then gradually bring down your body.

Aside from the particular yoga acts discussed above, the respiratory system can be protected from the dangers of different contaminations and ecological factors by incorporating a few herbs into everyday life. Three such Ayurvedic (ancient Indian medical system based on natural medicine) herbs have been shared below that proactively prevent sickness and lung damage by reinforcing the lung tissues.

- **Mulethi**

Instilled with strong antiviral, anti-inflammatory, antibacterial, and anti-allergic properties, Mulethi is very useful for treating problems in the throat, clearing sinus blockage, loosening mucus from the chest and nasal passage, lubricating irritated respiratory tract, and treating bronchitis and other asthmatic conditions. Daily use of this herb also reinforces lung tissues and improves lung well-being and function.

- **Vasaka**

The abundance of calming, anti-infection, and expectorant properties in Vasaka is a reflection of its utility in treating colds and influenza. It can also promote phlegm discharge, soothe bronchial inflammation, and lessen chest and nasal blockage due to sputum (a mixture of saliva and mucus).

- **Kalmegh**

This lovely ayurvedic herb is inherently honored with healing properties against microbial issues, contains cell reinforcement and stimulatory characteristics, and can play a crucial role in treating various kinds of fever, influenza, cold, and other respiratory problems.

Although yoga is one of the safest activities, make sure you take proper safety measures needed according to your health condition and check with a doctor or your medical practitioner as soon as possible if any issue arises or persists.

3.9 Yoga for Heart Disease

Yoga is a mind-body movement that includes traveling through a progression of body postures and breathing activities that can develop strength, adaptability, and stability and relax your mind. One of yoga's most clear advantages to the heart is its ability to relax the body and mind which can put the heart at ease. Emotional pressure and stress can cause a series of impacts on the body, including increased body chemicals like cortisol and adrenaline, which can result in the tightening and thinning of arteries leading to circulatory strain and issues. The deep breathing feature of yoga along with its calming effect can counterbalance this pressure, thus improving heart health.

Stress and depression can result in cardiovascular problems, such as coronary failure. As a general treatment plan, yoga can assist you in dealing with this pressure and stress since different poses of yoga help in bringing down your pulse, blood cholesterol, and glucose levels.

A scientific review has shown that daily yoga practice decreases the recurrence of atrial fibrillation episodes in patients with that condition. In another report, patients with cardiovascular disease who went through an eight-week yoga program showed improved cardiovascular health.

The act of yoga additionally can build strength, adaptability, and general endurance, making it an excellent practice for a healthy and satisfying lifestyle. The following are some yoga poses for a healthy heart.

- **Shoulder Stand Pose (Sarvangasana)**

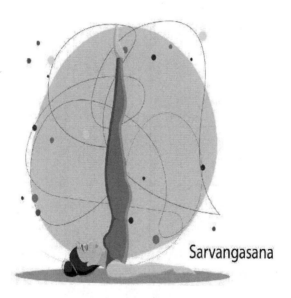

Sarvangasana

'Sarv' means all, 'Anga' means parts of a body, and 'asana' means act or pose. As the name suggests, this pose impacts all of the parts of your body and is exceptionally advantageous in keeping up with the physical and psychological well-being of a person. In this yoga pose, the entire body is balanced on the shoulders, which can calm the brain and relieve mild depression and stress that can lead to the improvement of heart health.

Lie on your back with hands beside your body. With one movement, lift your legs, bottom, and back up as high as possible and balance your entire weight on your shoulders. To maintain balance, use your hands and press them into the floor. Keep your legs firm and try not to press your neck into the floor. Hold this position for a few moments and take deep breaths. Let go when done. If you are finding this pose hard, try leaning against a wall. Once you have mastered this pose, move your hands closer to your back to make it even harder.

- **Warrior Pose (Virabhadrasana)**

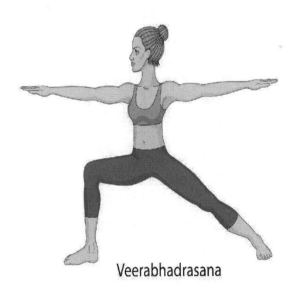

Veerabhadrasana

Warrior pose is a great pose to release stress, calm the mind, and control heart rate, all of which can play an important role in maintaining good heart health. It allows you to open up your chest and lungs, which encourages improved respiration and blood circulation.

Stand straight with your legs wide, separated by up to three to four feet. Turn your right foot out by 90 degrees and take a step to the right until you feel a deep stretch in your left leg. To maintain balance, turn your left foot in by around 15 degrees in the same direction. Keep your back straight and torso upright, with your arms either raised straight up or stretched out in the direction of your legs. Breathe deeply in this position and let go when tired.

There is much more in yoga besides the physical postures. The psychological angles are significant as well. Pranayama (breathing regulation) can be extremely valuable and assist with relaxing the sensory system, calming the breathing, and lowering the pulse or heart rate. Despite these amazing benefits, yoga should only be performed for up to fifty minutes (moderate yoga poses) each week, as it is anything but a high-impact action.

3.10 Yoga for Cancer

Yoga can assist individuals with malignant growth and cancer physically, emotionally, mentally, and spiritually. While it cannot battle malignant growth, yoga can alleviate some symptoms of cancer and its medicines. A few investigations have discovered that yoga may:

- *Ease malignant growth-related exhaustion*
- *Cause relaxation in the body*

- *Assist in the recovery from the medical procedures of malignant growth*
- *Decrease stress, nervousness, and pain*

Yoga is a mind-body practice that assists with lessening pressure and stress and improving adaptability and resilience. Some yoga poses are immensely beneficial for individuals with malignant growth. These include easy types of yoga poses such as Hatha yoga and supportive yoga, as these poses can assist in the treatment and make the symptoms more bearable.

Illness such as cancer can be emotionally, physically, and mentally upsetting. Since yoga is known to help with the emotional, physical, and mental needs of anyone who practices it, it can help with all these parts of malignant growth too. One investigation discovered that practicing a seven-week yoga routine increases the probability of creating healthy cancer-relieving chemicals by up to 65 percent. In addition, many experts have observed that the decrease in stress and pressure also improves personal satisfaction and could result in reduced pain intensity.

Cancer patients and survivors who are entirely new to yoga should talk with their doctors about the programs that might be appropriate to their condition. The following are three postures that can help cancer patients.

- **Legs Up the Wall Pose (Viparita Karani)**

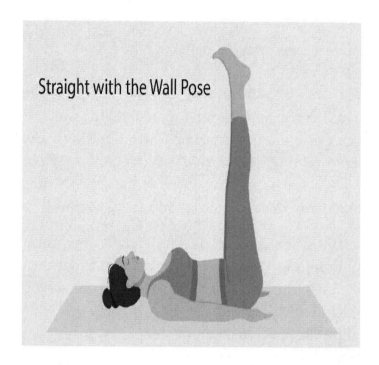

This posture can assist with combatting weakness either due to the symptoms of cancer or its treatment. First, lie next to a wall, with your feet touching the wall. Start to slide closer to the wall, taking small steps to move your feet up the wall as you use your arms to pull yourself closer to the wall. Your shoulders and head will lie on the floor while your legs stretch up the wall. Take deep breaths and remain in this position for a few minutes. Once you get comfortable with this pose, try raising your legs up without leaning against the wall.

- **Spinal Twist (Supta Matsyendrasana)**

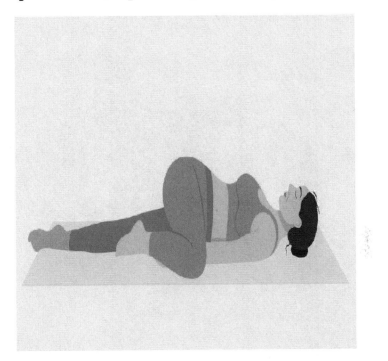

This posture can assist with spinal mobility and the absorption of food in the body. Begin by reclining on the ground with your limbs extended and your hands resting by your body. Draw your right knee closer to your chest and then cross it over your midline to place it on the left side of your body while keeping the left leg straight. Relax and take deep breaths, and then repeat on the other side.

- **Supine Bound Angle Pose (Supta Baddha Kosasana)**

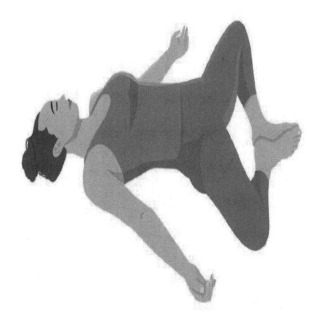

This pose can decrease weariness and stress in your body. Start by sitting down with your knees bent and the soles of your feet touching each other in front of your crotch. Gradually lie back, supporting yourself with your arms until your back is against the floor. Relax and breathe deeply with your arms out to your sides. Remain in this position for a few minutes and then repeat.

We all know that life is challenging and getting malignant growth or cancers and their treatments can add to these challenges considerably. In any case, as yogis, we are taught that suffering and pain are controllable and that we can change our pain into power with the realization that everything in life is for our strength.

3.11 Yoga for Bedtime

Practicing different yoga poses before sleeping is a method for letting go of all that is burdening you mentally or physically. Adding a yoga practice to your evening routine might improve the quality of your sleep. This is particularly useful for individuals who are struggling to rest, have sleep deprivation, or have limited time to rest. Continue reading to find out the different yoga poses you can try at home to improve your sleep.

- **Salutation Seal (Anjali Mudra)**

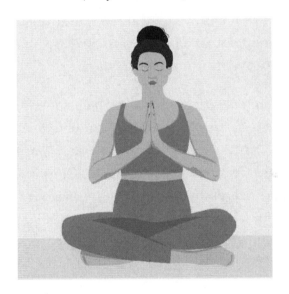

Take the hands together in supplication in front of the center of the chest, and pause for a minute to recognize the space around the heart. Remain in this position for ten minutes and think about three things that help you relax and breathe deeply.

- **Child's Pose (Balasana)**

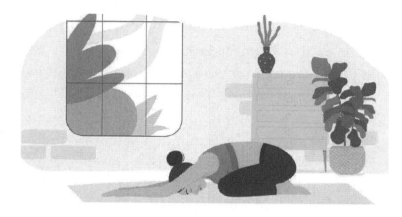

This yoga pose is for calming, quieting, and re-establishing the brain in the moment of stress. You can use this pose before sleeping to improve the quality of your sleep.

Start in a kneeling position with your feet under you. The knees can be separated or apart depending on what your body needs, and I suggest putting your hands in any position you feel relaxed in. Bend forward at your hips to bring your head down to the floor and rest your forehead between your hands. Stay in this position for about ten minutes (or more) and take deep breaths. You will feel relieved after this yoga pose and have a good sleep.

Yoga assists you in placing your body in a peaceful state, known as the relaxation reaction. This is something contrary to the instinctive response. Doing these yoga poses will assist you in many different ways such as helping you have a lower pulse and lower cortisol level, and easing stress-related issues, such as weight gain, uneasiness, and sleep deprivation. I am sure you would have learned a lot from this chapter, but it does not end here. Keep reading and learning further!

Chapter 4: Yoga as a Lifestyle

To some people, yoga is a type of activity performed to keep up with their physical well-being. However, practicing for physical well-being also comes with some mental and spiritual benefits, which is why, yoga can also improve a person's mental capacity and spiritual health.

Even though there are many different types of yoga, every one of them has something amazing, and acts as a scaffolding between physical and mental health, supporting and strengthing them both. It is a type of activity that, when performed correctly and regularly, can prompt new experiences in life. These experiences, originating from their inherent properties, urge the yogi to make them a part of their lifestyle.

Although the exact impact of yoga on the brain and body is yet to be completely confirmed, it is correct to say that yoga's relationship with relaxation and mindfulness is one of its extraordinary advantages. While performing yoga, one considers their presence, body, brain, and connection to the world around them, which can have a calming and relaxing impact.

It is also fair to contend that yoga is a type of specified meditation. By simply performing specific movements and postures with the feeling of care, the body goes into a meditative state in the same manner meditation takes it. Rather than feeling that one is forcefully taking their body through yoga, yoga becomes one with the needs of the body which is a fundamental part of this healthy routine. Unlike customary meditation and workout, yoga not only takes the status as a mix of meditation and workout but also enhances their individual benefits to improve the overall benefit to the user. Moreover, through dedication and regularity, yoga can significantly influence the lifestyle of an individual for the better, which only improves with time.

The vital distinction between the people who perform yoga as an activity and those who treat it as a lifestyle is the utilization of yoga's experiences in their everyday life. While on the mat, the advantages are clear, and one feels over the moon after the practice ends. But, outside of the mat, the advantages are much broader such as better mood, reduced stress, calmness of mind, better decision making, and overall stronger body which supports resilience.

Yoga puts the yogi in an uplifted state, where what is normally disregarded becomes immensely significant and irrefutable: an enthusiasm for one's presence as a physical and mental being. Yoga provides a life far away from machines and prompts adequate and in-depth reflection of one's inward and public life. As far as some might be concerned, these considerations result from both yoga as an activity and a lifestyle, however, for people who consider it as a lifestyle, the results are far greater and form a bedrock of events that stack up on each other to provide continuous benefits.

It can be said that all yogis maintain a yogic lifestyle to some extent by consistently performing yoga that prompts the realization of the specific advantages that yoga yields. Achieving these benefits and results of yoga can fundamentally modify one's everyday life such as changing one's relationships with others, moral and mindset changes, and potential dietary changes (like adopting vegetarianism). Through yoga, yogis experience an unending series of changes to one's lifestyle and almost everyone will agree that many of these progressions and changes are considered to be positive.

It is completely plausible that a more extravagant daily routine can be experienced by taking on yoga as a lifestyle. Remember, with its experience and application, one can easily enhance many factors of their life. Yoga can be the foundation of a beautiful lifestyle and the following are some of the lifestyle and health issues that can be cured with yoga.

4.1 Yoga for Weight Loss

Yoga movement has helped many individuals effortlessly shed a few pounds. Yoga for weight reduction is an actual theme within the world of yoga, however, as many individuals acknowledge, yoga alone cannot help in weight reduction. Yoga combined with good dieting has proved to be valuable for a large number of people as it assists them with getting fit and keeping their minds and body healthy. It changes the way one cares for and connects with their body and prompts them to start looking for healthy food options instead of gorging on unhealthy food that can build loads of fat in their body.

Losing weight has two significant components, smart dieting, and exercise, both of which can be achieved by practicing yoga. Yoga is not just about a few poses that improve your flexibility and mental health; it brings more advantages, such as weight reduction, good spiritual health, relaxation, and calmness of mind among many others. Stress can devastatingly affect your brain and body as it can manifest itself as torment, nervousness, sleeping disorders, and the inability to focus. Occasionally, stress can also lead to weight gain. Since yoga is known to assist people in controlling their stress, it can help individuals get in shape and maintain their physical and psychological well-being.

Yoga will not bring one's weight down rapidly as most of its poses are relatively less strenuous. However, there are certain poses within yoga that can be more effective in weight reduction called power yoga poses. These poses of yoga focus on building flexibility, strength, endurance, and size. You will definitely see your weight fall when your body becomes acquainted with these Asanas and postures.

Power yoga is a novel kind of yoga that has its basic formations in Ashtanga yoga. These Asanas create hotness inside the body and augment your perseverance, making you stronger and more versatile, and freeing you from your tensions and stress. Ashtanga yoga is a series of strength-building poses that engage and activate every part of your body.

Most power yoga begins with Sun Salutation (Surya Namaskara), which can be used as a warm-up before starting the actual yoga session. Following are the different power yoga poses that you can start attempting!

- **Sun Salutation Pose (Surya Namaskar)**

This is a power yoga pose for weight reduction that can help people ranging from amateurs to even specialists. It is a series of 12 poses which should ideally be done first thing in the morning for up to 12 rounds.

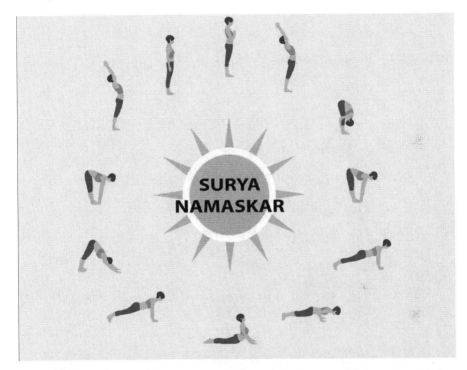

- *Step 1: Pranamasana (Prayer Pose): Stand straight with feet together and your weight equally distributed on your feet. Relax your shoulders and expand your chest with your arms resting on your sides. As you breathe in, raise your arms up from the sides and join the palms of your hands to perform a Namaskar (a traditional Indian greeting where palms are joined in front of the face or chest as a sign of respect).*

- *Step 2: Hastauttanasana (Raised arms pose): Stretch your arms up and back and curve backward to stretch the whole body from fingertips to heels.*

- *Step 3: Hasta Padasana (Hand to Foot pose): Bend forward at your hips as you breathe out to touch your feet. To feel a deeper stretch, try to touch your head to your knees.*

- *Step 4: Ashwa Sanchalanasana (Equestrian pose): Move your right leg back as you bring your right knee to the ground. Rest your left foot directly behind your side as you place your palms on the floor and look up.*

- *Step 5: Dandasana (Stick Pose): Bring your left leg back to your right leg while breathing out. Lift your hips off of the floor with your arms perpendicular to the floor, keeping your neck, back, and legs in a straight line.*

- *Step 6: Ashtanga Nmaskara (Salute with Eight Parts): Touch the ground with your feet, knees, chest, chin, and palms by bringing your body down to the ground level, with your hip slightly raised off of the floor.*

- *Step 7: Bhuangasana (Cobra pose): bring your hips to the floor, lifting your chest and face up by pressing your palms into the floor and looking up, as discussed in section 3.4.*

- *Step 8: Parvatasana (Grounded Mountain Pose): Let your head fall between your arms as you lift your hips to the ceiling to form a mountain or an inverted "V" pose while breathing.*

- **Side Stretch Pose (Parsvottanasana)**

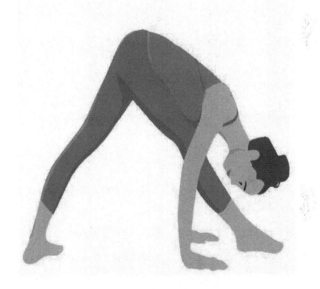

This yoga position can be performed either in the morning or in the evening on an empty stomach. Begin by standing tall with your hands at your sides, palms down. Step your left foot to the left and slowly bend over at the hip towards your left foot, as if you are attempting to touch the floor with your hands. Strive to keep your knees straight. Hold this posture for fifteen seconds before switching to the other side. For desired outcomes, engage in this routine for ten minutes a day.

- **Wind Releasing Posture (Pawanmuktasana)**

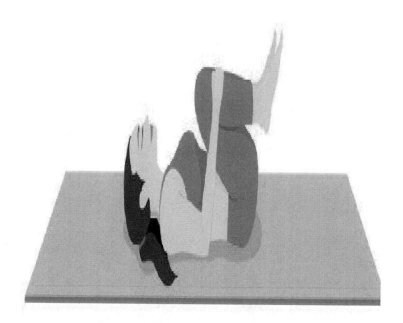

To effectively lose weight, make sure you have an empty stomach when you practice this position either in the morning or evening. Start by lying on your back and positioning your hands on both sides. Then, bring your knees up and raise your legs towards your chest, using your hands to apply pressure on your legs against your chest. Stay in this position for about fifteen seconds before repeating the process. Set aside ten to fifteen minutes daily to perform this posture and achieve your weight loss goals.

- **Eagle Pose (Garudasana)**

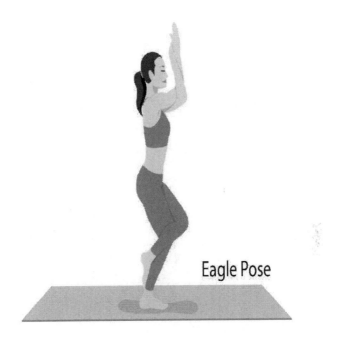

Eagle Pose

The best way to practice this posture is on an empty stomach either in the morning or evening. Stand straight with hands on either side of the body. Balance your body weight on your right leg by lifting your left leg up and marginally bending your knees. Wrap your left leg over your right leg and then raise your arms above, with your elbows parallel to the ground and palms pressed against each other. Remain in this position for ten seconds and then, come back into the resting position. Practice this pose multiple times a day for up to ten minutes at a time.

Yoga, an Indian way of mind and body revival, has enormous advantages for all from individuals who are stout and need to shed some weight to individuals who need to relax as it is a deep-rooted treatment for a healthy body and a calm psyche.

Yoga leads to weight reduction when combined with an excellent and healthy diet, which will be discussed in the following chapters. Read on!

4.2 The Benefits of Having a Strong Core

Often, people prioritize having aesthetically pleasing abs over building a strong core. However, developing core strength offers a range of valuable benefits such as improved balance, reduced back pain, and enhanced mental health.

To clarify, your core is not just located near your navel. While many individuals assume the core solely consists of the abdominal muscles, it also encompasses the muscles in your pelvis, mid and lower back, and even your hip muscles. These muscles work in unison to support your spine and head in a neutral position.

Visualize your core as a solid foundation that upholds your entire body, providing a stable center of gravity whether you are stationary or in motion. Just as a ballet dancer centers themselves to maintain balance during turns, you rely on your core strength for everyday activities such as walking, sitting, exercising, or performing any physical movement. Since almost all of the body's movements start from the core, enhancing and increasing its strength will do wonders for everyone while maintaining a healthy spinal cord. Keep reading to learn about more of the benefits of a strong core!

- **Improves posture**

Performing core exercises engages all the muscles from your upper to lower body and from front to back. This helps you maintain an upright posture with well-aligned limbs. By improving the positioning of your spine, you can reduce the risk of herniation in your core and degeneration in your vertebrae. Not only that but better balance resulting from good posture can also help open up your respiratory tract and make breathing easier.

- **Better athletic performance**

Core strength is essential for nearly every sport. For instance, runners can prevent their legs and arms from tiring by incorporating core exercises into their routine. Rowers rely heavily on their core as they paddle, with a stronger core allowing them to pull with greater speed and power. Baseball pitchers generate power for their throws from both their arms and core. Therefore, improving your core strength can undoubtedly boost your athletic performance.

- **Eases up back pain**

Studies indicate that individuals with weak core muscles are more susceptible to spinal pain and injuries due to inadequate spinal support. To alleviate body pains, enhance resilience and strength, and promote stability, core exercises and workouts like yoga can be effective. Moreover, these activities can also reinforce spinal function and decrease the risk of spinal injury.

- **Safer everyday movement**

Performing daily activities such as standing upright, lifting objects, sitting, bending down, playing with children, and climbing stairs can become effortless with a strong core. Strengthening your core enhances muscle control, preventing certain muscles from becoming overburdened.

- **Improves balance and stability**

Poor stability and balance, which may result from lower body inadequacy, spinal injuries, or neurological deficiencies, can greatly impact daily tasks. Research has shown that core strength improvement can enhance balance and stability, thus facilitating everyday activities.

Unlike strength-based exercises that target individual muscle groups, core workouts engage multiple muscle groups throughout the body. Yoga, in particular, can be an excellent way to strengthen your core, provided that the poses or positions you practice focus on core muscles. If you are new to these activities, expect to feel some cramping in your lower and upper back, and lower body the day after the workout. This discomfort is your core muscles responding to the workout and building up.

It's advisable to spend a few minutes each day engaging in core-supporting exercises. Although it may be challenging initially, persisting with it will yield worthwhile benefits and results. Through core exercises, you will experience improvements in how you look, feel, and move throughout the day.

4.3 Yoga Routines to Do with a Partner

It is so natural to fall into relationship ruts. When you are completely in love with your life partner, you do loads of things together such as eating, going to the movies and parks, or just spending time together as you watch your favorite TV show. Of course, it is lovely, but it can get very boring at times. Adding a little change to your routine can reignite the spark with your partner and yoga could be exactly what you need in those times.

The following yoga poses for you to practice with your partner can be somewhat difficult at the start, but, their results can be extraordinary for beginners. You do not need to be a yoga master to try these poses; you just need to make sure to consistently pay attention to your body, concentrate on your breathing, and do nothing that can injure you. What you need more is to chuckle and have an amazing time with your life partner. Check the following poses and start practicing today!

- **Partner Seated Twist Pose**

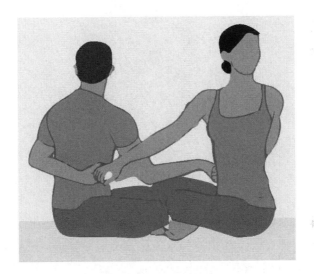

Start in a seated position with your legs crossed and your backs leaning against one another. Place your hands on your thighs or knees and let yourself feel and associate with your partner. As you breathe in, place your arms over your head, extending the spine as you reach up. Breathe out and tilt to the right towards your partner's left knee and try to grab it with your right hand. Your partner should move to the opposite side. Hold each other in the position for three to five breaths and then let go. Repeat on the opposite side for a few turns as you build your connection with your partner.

- **Partner Breathing Pose**

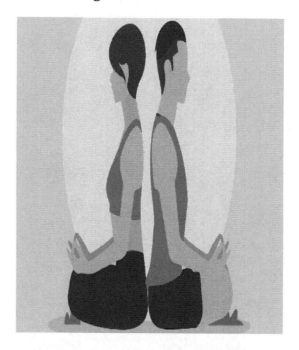

Start in a seated position with legs crossed and your backs leaning against one another in Burmese Position (Sukhasana) as discussed in section 3.2 of this book.

As you allow yourself to feel and associate with your partner, start to see how your breathing aligns with each other as you breathe in and out and how the back of the spine feels against your partner's. Start to breathe alternatively with your partner, so as you breathe in, your partner breathes out, and so forth. Practice for three to five minutes to really connect with your partner.

- **Twin Trees Pose**

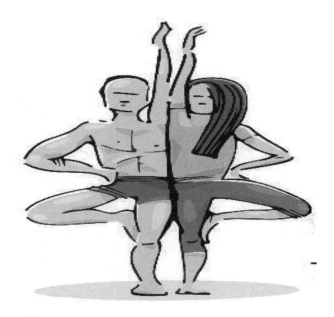

Stand close to one another side by side. Start to move weight onto your inner foot and bend your outer leg to place it on your inner as you lean against your partner. Let your partner do the same. Place your outer arm on your waist or join the palms of your outer hand with your partner's outer hand in front of your chests. With the inner arms, either place them on each other's back to hold each other, or raise them straight up and press your palms against each other. Balance for five to seven minutes. Repeat the process.

- **Partner Forward Fold Pose**

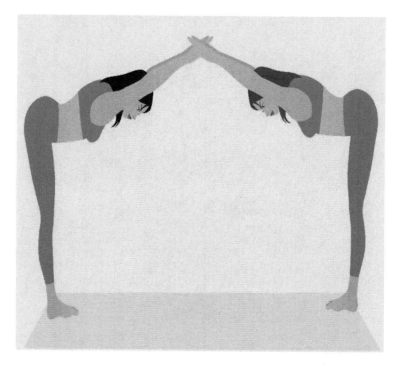

Start by facing each other in a standing position with your feet straight under the hips. At that point, breathe in, raise your arms over your head, and start to pivot forward at the hips until your hands meet with your partner's. Gradually begin to move farther away from your partner so your arms are leveled with the floor. Hold for five to seven minutes as you feel a deep stretch in your back and legs and then let go.

- **Seated Forward-Fold Partner Pose**

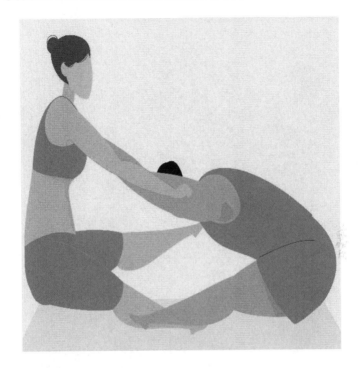

From a seated position facing one another, stretch the legs out to a wide "V" shape, with kneecaps facing straight up and the bottoms of your feet pressed against your partner's feet. Extend your arms toward one another and hold each other's hands. As you breathe in, extend up through the spine. As you breathe out, one individual folds forward from the hips while the other partner continues to sit back, keeping their spine and arms straight. Remain in the posture for five to seven minutes and come back into the seated position again. Repeat with the other partner now folding forward.

- **Partner Boat Pose**

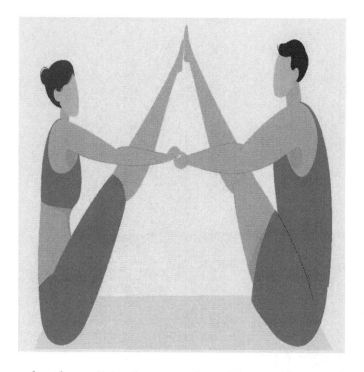

Facing each other, sit in the seated position with your legs fully extended and the soles of your feet pressed against your partner's. Extend your arms and grab each other's hands gently. While keeping the soles of your feet pressed against each other and holding each other's hand, start to move closer to each other and bend your legs at your knees while raising your feet off of the ground.

To make it easier at first, try bending and lifting one leg at a time. Lift your chests up and extend your spines as much as possible. Hold yourself in this position for five to seven minutes and take deep breaths.

- **Partner Squat**

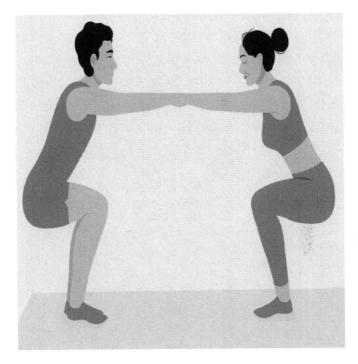

Stand facing each other with your feet shoulder-distance apart. Hold each other's hands or forearms, then slowly lower into a squat, keeping your backs straight and your knees directly over your toes. Hold the squat for a few breaths, then slowly stand up. This pose can help to build leg strength and improve balance, while also promoting a sense of connection and teamwork with your partner.

Remember to move slowly and mindfully, and to stop immediately if you feel any pain or discomfort. It's also a good idea to have a chair or wall nearby for support if needed. With any of the yoga poses that are practiced as a couple, communication and trust are the keys to success, so be sure to communicate clearly with your partner and listen to their feedback and needs.

After completing these poses, come to a neutral position lying close to one another on your backs, and place your hands on each other's hands delicately. Allow your body to relax with your eyes shut. Feel the closeness of your partner and your relationship with them and relax in this position for three to five minutes before finishing your training. Get to know your partner and yourself better with these team-driven postures. Hope you both love these poses!

Chapter 5: Personal Evolution

The expression "personal evolution," like "care" and "otherworldliness," has become a popular one, so much so that it is at risk of losing its power and significance. According to yoga, personal evolution is more than just a personal development project or a goal to build new habits. It is a progressive and long-lasting change in how we connect with ourselves and the world.

Personal evolution encompasses the development of all aspects of our personhood, including relations with ourselves and others. It also includes a sense of otherworldly association, scholarly and innovative development, acknowledgment, and support of our physical bodies. Finally, personal evolution means the ability to explore our changing feelings with empathy and a healthy measure of distance.

If personal evolution appears lengthy and challenging, keep in mind that development in one space leads to growth in another. The pieces of ourselves and our lives are inextricably linked. One small change results in what is referred to as a "positive vertical winding"—an opposite cascading type of influence that promotes flourishing.

Remember that the journey of personal evolution may begin with a conscious, deliberate start, but it does not end there. It is a long-term practice. So, remember to practice, practice, and keep practicing! We can never attain perfection as there will always be room for improvement and growth every step of the way. So put yourself to the test of living: feel what it is like to try something new, see what happens when your master a new pose, and practice not being overly attached to the outcome. That is how we rewire our brains and gain new perspectives on how we see and experience life.

Yoga and meditation are two of the most effective and widely available tools when it comes to revitalizing our minds. According to research, these practices change the brain, improving and strengthening regions associated with prosperity and decreasing activity in the amygdala, the part of the brain associated with fear and reactivity.

A research scholar investigated the impact of ordinary cherishing and considering thoughts on people's everyday experiences and discovered that they increased positive feelings such as love, euphoria, appreciation, happiness, trust, pride, interest, and entertainment. Thus, these feelings are linked to increases in various individual properties, features, and characteristics, including careful consideration, self-acknowledgment, good relationships, and excellent physical health. So, if you are looking for a place to start, yoga is a perfect practice to create all these positive changes.

What happens on the yoga mat should carry over into our interactions with others if we want to evolve personally. Being in a relationship with your body is a profound yoga practice and being human entails being associated. Therefore, we have to carry our learnings from the mat to our associations and relationships, regardless of whether we develop a habit of being alone on the mat.

Connections become groundbreaking when we put our necks out there by being honest and open. There is no guarantee that things will work out how we want them to when we maintain truth in our relationships. Many of your loved ones may accept the reality and appreciate you for being honest; many would not. But, it is important to recognize that truth and honesty are fundamental to a long-lasting relationship and that positive changes come from being straightforward, open, and able to get and be affected by what comes from that validity.

A relationship with yourself is also essential to the path of personal evolution. It is vital to figure out how to find peace within, as well as to acknowledge and respect our identity. This includes paying close attention to our physical bodies through proper nutrition, exercise, and self-love.

One slight shift practiced over a long time is one way to complete the course of change. That could be as simple as going out more often, spending a couple of moments every day to inhale deeply and intentionally as you focus on your breathing to relax and calm your mind, interacting with people you care about, or incorporating imaginative and creative thinking slots into your schedules, whatever is best for you. Innovation means living to our full potential and it is important to note that everything we do exemplifies a creative decision.

Self-sympathy, care, and love may be the most important things to learn on this path of personal evolution. Development cannot be linear; it comes in waves, pushing ahead, pulling back, and then pushing ahead again, similar to meditation, where every breath, every second, is an opportunity to focus on being present and mindful and enjoy the benefits of that mindfulness. Patience is required in development; a seed planted today does not grow into a tree the next day, it does so only over time, at its own pace and desire.

5.1 Motivating Yourself to Practice Yoga Regularly

I do a lot of yoga. I do it regardless of whether I am traveling, busy, or exhausted. Most people frequently ask me how I manage to keep myself motivated. My response is that it is a habit I have developed and enjoy. So, just as our parents taught us to brush our teeth regularly, I taught myself to do yoga regularly. There is no point in doing anything wellness-related if it is only for a day, a week, or a month. If you want any wellness-related effort to provide long-term benefits, you must do it regularly. It could be 10 minutes a day or 60 minutes, but it is consistency that will help you the most. So, fellas, if you are looking for motivation to start practicing yoga regularly, then I have a lot of advice for you. Just keep reading!

- **Attend a yoga class**

Do you have a lot of family responsibilities? If so, joining a yoga studio may be your best option. Although it may appear counterproductive, it may be the primary method by which you will escape your "work" zone and enter your yoga zone. Your family tasks will present themselves regularly and your need to learn how to coordinate them better so that you expend less energy and time doing them and have some left for later to work on your self-love and care through yoga. Some of you will say that this is more difficult than one might expect. Correct, but this is something you must do to begin a yoga practice.

- **Set aside time for yoga and treat it as a daily ritual**

"How would you even set aside time to do yoga regularly with a baby?" This, my friends, is the most compelling reason why some of us do not practice yoga regularly and others do. It will not be easy to set aside time and stick to it regularly unless you make it a daily habit. If you work or have young children to care for, or both, realize that you are not alone. Everyone struggles with the number of hours they have in a day. The key here is to think about how you can be more efficient with your time. Can you find some time for yoga, or other self-care routines, by giving up things that are not assisting you in reaching your goals? For example, you might need to reduce your TV time, long phone calls, or an hour of rest. Try it for a week and see how you feel.

Assuming you live alone - fantastic, this will most likely be less difficult for you. When you save yourself some time, notify your companion, children, and other relatives. Inform them that it is essential for you and that they should allow you to have this time to yourself. If you have friends or family members who like to drop by unannounced, ensure they are aware, so they do not interfere with your yoga time.

- **Set objectives**

This one is for you if you enjoy staring off into space or looking at photographs or your phones for hours before realizing you don't have much time left to complete your chores or work on your personal development and care. Do you find the process of defining objectives exhausting? Honestly, this can be a lot of fun. Before I was regular with my training, I saw yoga pictures and wished I could do some of the postures. It was only when I set an objective that I realized that I needed to figure out how to do different poses rather than just look at them. The yoga Asana that got me started was the vertical bow. Although it took me months to perfect it, the progress I saw during that time got me hooked.

Nobody ever starts anything wellness-related without a goal in mind. Many people need to start yoga to achieve a specific wellness, adaptability, or strength level. Or maybe they need to lose a couple of pounds. Ask yourself what your goal is; perhaps it is to develop the strength to perform a specific asana, or just feel more confident in yourself. Try not to pass judgment on yourself based on your goal. Try not to let others judge you, regardless of whether they do, do not let it affect you.

- **Begin slowly and take small steps**

Allow your first few days to be slow and delicate. Whether you are practicing yoga at home or joining a studio, I recommend you start with beginner poses for the first few days. You may be discouraged from returning to training if the first day is too much to handle or complex. Also, it would help if you cared for your body and did not overly exhaust your muscles.

- **Track your progress**

Seeing your progress is the most consistent source of motivation to practice any kind of wellness-related activity. Take note of how your body moves and feels. Keep a mental record of your psychological edge. Try not to push yourself too far beyond your comfort zone at first, but pay attention to where it is. Determine how long or how many breaths you can hold a specific yoga asana. By keeping a track of your progress, you can adjust your objectives and pace as you move through different levels of yoga poses.

- **Select your favorite pair of yoga pants**

If you have ever worked in an office, you have probably seen the inspiring power of dressing with a specific goal. No, you do not have to be in a client-facing job, but when you dress in new office attire, you will notice how you feel more confident and how people take you more seriously. It is important to keep in mind the persuasive power of seemingly unimportant or insignificant things. So go ahead; indulge yourself in wearing your comfortable yoga pants. There is no need to concentrate on examining them for their distinct features but rather on how you feel when you wear them. Obviously, bonus points if the yoga pants make you look and feel attractive!

- **Find and keep things that inspire you in sight**

I tell everyone I know about this tip because it has always worked for me: to accomplish something, find out what is motivating you to do it, and keep it as close to you as possible throughout the day. It could be a statement, a picture of a yoga pose, or simply your mat - the idea is to keep your inspiration visible. It could be your phone's or computer's screensaver. If you are embarrassed about other people seeing it, you can keep it hidden, but definitely choose a picture that helps you remember yoga and reminds you why you started practicing it in the first place.

- **Reward yourself for practicing**

Praise small victories and reward yourself for showing up. Now is not the time to get carried away and reward yourself with something that will hinder your advancement. Instead, clean up, order a hearty meal from the grill, watch your favorite show, or talk about it to your friends. Do what your time allows you to ensure your psyche can handle it. It does not have to be large, but it should be hearty and warm and should fill you up!

The fact that you are reading this book implies that you are looking for motivation to get back into your yoga routine or to start a new daily routine. Try not to wait for another week or a month before you start. Start today!

5.2 Self-Analyzing and Self-Corrections to Get Fit

Benjamin Franklin, who lived over quite a while back, utilized monitoring techniques to keep tabs on his development toward the 13 objectives he had set for himself. He accepted that the logging system extended his mindfulness and supported his endeavors to change his way of behaving. He stated: "I was astonished to find myself full of deficiencies than I had thought of before," and also said, "yet I had the fulfillment of seeing them reduce."

Today, many successful individuals utilize similar strategies to accomplish more and perform better. First-class competitors, for instance, regularly keep monitoring logs of their exhibitions and practices and of the elements that add to their specific goals. Research affirms that recording parts of progress and behavior toward objectives — a technique many analysts call self-monitoring — upgrades your progress to making an assortment of life changes. Self-monitoring has become a powerful apparatus for athletic performance, scholarly accomplishment, and nurturing abilities; in clinical circumstances, self-observing has been displayed to support reducing weight, smoking, problematic conduct, nail gnawing, and even procrastination! When joined with objective setting and other methods that change conduct, self-monitoring is a straightforward, yet integral asset that wellness experts use to assist clients in accomplishing their goals and more.

- **Self-monitoring is effective**

For a plethora of reasons, self-monitoring develops performance. Whenever individuals perform well, it gives them a little fulfilling reward by keeping tabs on their development and giving themselves a "passing mark" which can boost their sense of joy and commitment. When they are not performing, by giving themselves a "poor grade," individuals can use self-monitoring as a suggestion to rethink and reevaluate their approach. For instance, an individual might miss an exercise one day because of commitments at work or home. Instead of being tough on themselves, they should devise a methodology to assist them with adhering to the system. It could be as simple as getting up an hour earlier and doing the activity then, or they compose the exercise in their life's book and honor it as an important ritual.

Self-checking helps people in keeping away from unrealistic and counterproductive thinking, such as beliefs that often prompt the "compounding phenomenon": experiencing a minor difficulty, marking oneself as a "disappointment," and permitting that little pass to accelerate into a significant backslide and add up to imploding an individual. Moreover, self-checking will generally neutralize the habit of neglecting progress.

Self-monitoring also makes it hard for people to justify slow advancement or overlook mishaps by driving them to be responsible and accountable to themselves. Consider this individual's insight, who involved self-observing as a component of their weight reduction program: "When I was keeping records of the foods I ate in a day, there were days when I didn't record anything. First, I had to remind myself why I was monitoring my food **intake and why I had been slacking off. Then, I had to face my physical sentiments. Did I need to quit eating excessively or not? I concluded I did, so I constrained myself to ignore the justifications** for why I did not need to quit eating excessively. That functioned admirably, and I immediately returned to keeping records regularly."

Self-monitoring makes "corrections" a lot easy. Individuals who keep tabs on their development toward their eating and exercise objectives, for instance, often find they are encountering "end of the week snowballs" — gaining consistent headway during the week yet permitting minor slips to accelerate into some days. With this information, self-monitoring can help them try harder to practice at the end of the week and also to prepare quality suppers at home instead of eating out.

Imagine, you see growing trend lines and charts of your personal progress on a spreadsheet. Sounds motivating, right? Well, you are not alone. Many find that consistently rising trend lines demonstrating one's growth and progress are more rousing and reasonable than columns of numbers. So try creating charts of your progress to see how it's trending to motivate yourself more. You will not profit from exercise information on the off chance that it is just accessible on your clipboard or in an incorporated document. They should be in front of you consistently and presented in a motivating way.

The gist is that you will be more committed and stick to a new routine when you monitor your progress. You start by monitoring controllable elements like exercise length and exersion level instead of "result measures" like weight, circulatory strain, muscle-to-fat ratio, or prescription necessities. I am sure you can make effective use of the information above!

Chapter 6: Diet Modifications with Yoga

Practicing yoga and maintaining a healthy eating routine is not relatively as straightforward as you would suspect. No one has mentioned a yoga diet since ancient yogic texts like Patanjali's Yoga Sutra and Bhagavad Gita.

An Ayurvedic diet has been drilled for millennia in ancient India and is followed by numerous yogis. This eating regimen is based on Ayurvedic medication, which helps the individuals who follow it connect more with nature and their surroundings. So, how about we investigate this Ayurvedic diet?

The expression "Ayurveda" is derived from two Sanskrit words: "Ayus", which means life span or imperativeness, and "Veda", which means intelligence or science. Therefore, Ayurveda signifies "the study of life and life span." Ayurveda has existed since the time of the Vedic sacred texts, old Hindu texts that covered Hindu culture and history dating back 5000 years. It is a logical way to deal with the medication that utilizes homegrown herbs, yoga, and dietary changes to treat illness and improve well-being. By combining sustenance with lifestyle changes, the Ayurvedic diet helps individuals in staying healthy or heal from illnesses. Ayurveda is a comprehensive concept that helps deal with well-being and focuses on sickness and forestalling it. Understanding your body and its requirements permits you to make a better and more joyful lifestyle for yourself.

The fundamental distinction between an Ayurvedic diet and a normal diet is that in an Ayurvedic diet, you eat as per your mind-body type, also known as "Dosha", which describes your unique personality, physical nature, and tendencies. Pitta (dosha of water and fire elements), Vata (space and air dosha), and Kapha (dosha of earth and water) are the three doshas. Eating as indicated by your predominant dosha helps keep your body in balance. If you are struggling to understand or figure out your dosha, I would encourage you to counsel an Ayurvedic specialist, who will be able to guide you on the best food varieties to eat in light of your predominant dosha.

> **Would it be a good idea for you to follow an Ayurvedic diet?**

Regardless of your dosha type, the Ayurvedic diet suggests eating food varieties that are great for you and helps you keep away from those that are bad for you. This incorporates avoiding processed foods, low-quality food, and anything containing additives, fake flavors, and added substances.

Vegetables (particularly salad greens), rice, whole grains, and beans are all important components of an Ayurvedic diet. What food types would it be a good idea for you to avoid while following an Ayurvedic diet, you may ask? Most followers of the Ayurvedic diet will say caffeine, dairy items, gluten-containing food varieties like bread and pasta, and red meat are everything to stay away from. It must be noted that this is not a vegan diet, however, it encourages eating less meat than numerous other diet plans.

6.1 The Importance of Diet with Yoga

What we eat affects not only our physical well-being but also our emotions and mental well-being. Therefore, yoga does not categorize food as proteins, carbohydrates, or fats but instead divides it into three different categories based on their impact on the body and mind: Sattva or Sattvic diet (linked to knowledge and purity), Rajas or Rajasic diet (linked to ignorance and darkness), and Tamas or Tamasic (linked to attachment and strong emotions).

- **Sattvic diet**

Sattvic food types are pure and nurturing, promoting well-being, mental clarity, strength, and relaxation. These include leafy foods, vegetables and herbs, honey, whole grains, nuts, and seeds. The key here is that these foods should be naturally grown, naturally obtained, and free of added substances and additives. An added benefit of these food sources is that they are simple to prepare. Eating slowly, admirably, and thoroughly enjoying each bite is also considered Sattvic.

- **Tamasic diet**

A Tamasic diet in today's world is what we call "Junk Food"; it is neither beneficial to the mind nor the body. This diet includes food sources that can be stale, under and over-ripe, rotten or fermented, and tasteless. Tamasic food varieties can be challenging to digest, making you feel bloated. They can also lower the body's immunity, affect the nervous system, and make one greedy or angry which is why a tamasic diet is linked to over-indulgence.

- **Rajasic diet**

Rajasic food varieties are fresh and nutritious and promote an abundance of energy in the body. These food types are activating and stimulating, and energize every system of the body. However, an excess of these foods can cause a mental restlessness, rage, hyperactivity, and anxiety. Some of the foods in this category include meat, fish, chicken, coffee, dark tea desserts, chocolate, spices or chilies, a few flavorings, and eggs. Eating in a hurry is also considered Rajasic.

In addition to eating the proper type of food, it is critical to consume an adequate amount of food. Over-indulgence induces dormancy, whereas not eating enough may lead to insufficient sustenance. Most of the time, we are aware that our stomach is full but are enticed by the taste buds which leads to overeating. The ideal food proportion cannot be measured in cups or grams; however, if we pay close attention to our bodies, we will know when to stop!

We may eat the right kind of food in the right amount, but if we are inconsistent with our timings, the entire framework goes for a toss and harms the body's everyday temperament. As a result, it is critical to eat food that is both usual and standard and eaten at regular intervals and frequency.

It is believed that the mental state of the person who is cooking or eating influences their food. For example, the energy in food prepared by someone angry will be lower than that of someone who cooked it with feelings of affection, satisfaction, and appreciation. Standing nearby and listening to soothing music while cooking and eating can help keep the Prana (life power energy) in the food.

Yoga also suggests a more personalized diet based on the concept of our constitution. Food that is beneficial to one person may be detrimental to another. Therefore, it is best to consult with a doctor to determine which foods are essential for you and which ones should be avoided. Nonetheless, it is undoubtedly beneficial to give some thought to the food we eat; as old Indian texts say "We are what we eat!"

6.2 Optimal One-Week Diet Plan

The food we eat essentially affects what we look like and how we feel. Our daily activity plays a significant role; however, nourishment affects our wellness too, as confirmed through research. Eating food as medicine has become a well-being improvement subject that focuses on having quality food as an essential wellness objective. We feel better and more joyful when a good diet becomes a part of our lifestyle.

Practicing good eating habits can assist us with losing weight while retaining muscle, feeling more sure and confident, and bringing down sickness. As per various investigations, the main part of our workout regimes is good food consumption. Supplemented food sources, or "superfoods," contain lean proteins, good carbs, and fats that are fundamental for our well-being. In addition, superfoods are high in nutrients, minerals, and cancer prevention agents and low in calories.

Healthy food assists our bodies in battling sickness by lessening irritation. Numerous diseases are supposed to be brought about due to irritation. Cancer prevention agents tracked down in mixed greens and vegetables, for instance, assist with safeguarding our cells from extreme harm. In addition, some superfoods contain intensifiers that support our digestion, permitting us to consume fat more productively. For example, red peppers contain capsaicin that improves metabolism and burns more energy and fat.

As you can see, good food is essential for a healthy life, and combining it with yoga can add a lot more benefits to your lifestyle. I have designed a one-week plan to help you initiate your diet routine at home. First, follow the meal plan routine below and then make amendments to your diet according to your choices.

Day 1:	
Breakfast: Black current and kale smoothie	186 kcalories
Lunch: Parmesan Chicken and Spinach	402 kcalories
Snack: Melon and Grape Juice	125 kcalories
Dinner: Aromatic chicken with salsa	434 kcalories
Total	**1147 kcalories**

Day 2:	
Breakfast: Green tea smoothie	183 kcalories
Lunch: Miso marinated cod with stir-fried greens	450 kcalories
Snack: Strawberry cucumber juice	192 kcalories
Dinner: Beef Arabiata	402 kcalories
Total	**1227 kcalories**

Day 3:	
Breakfast: Date and Walnut Oatmeal	350 kcalories
Lunch: Lemon kale chicken pasta	620 kcalories
Snack: Black current and kale smoothie	186 kcalories
Dinner: Sesame Chicken salad	304 kcalories
Total	**1460 kcalories**

Day 4:	
Breakfast: Blueberry pancakes	509 kcalories
Lunch: Baked salmon with mint dressing	420 kcalories
Snack: Green Juice	143 kcalories
Dinner: Turmeric chicken and Salad with lime	416 kcalories
Total	**1488 kcalories**

Day 5:	
Breakfast: Oat and Berry Acai Bowl	501 kcalories
Lunch: Lamb Butternut Squash and Date Tagine	244 kcalories
Snack: Fruit Salad	172 kcalories
Dinner: Pot Chicken and Kale Curry	486 kcalories
Total	**1403 kcalories**

Day 6:	
Breakfast: *Smoked Salmon Omelette*	*349 kcalories*
Lunch: *Chicken Coronation Salad*	*102 kcalories*
Snack: *Choc Chip Granola*	*244 kcalories*
Dinner: *Spicy Chickpea Stew with Baked Potatoes*	*352 kcalories*
Total	**1047 kcalories**

Day 7:	
Breakfast: *Shakshuka*	*184 kcalories*
Lunch: *Kale and Red Onion Dhal with Buckwheat*	*420 kcalories*
Snack: *Chocolate Bites*	*272 kcalories*
Dinner: *Kale, Edamame, and Tofu Curry*	*344 kcalories*
Total	**1220 kcalories**

Always remember to cook your food at home if you can or at least try to cook most of the times, if not all the time. Eat healthily and follow the section below for some amazing diet tips to be followed along with your regular yoga sessions.

6.3 Different Eating Tips and Techniques to Boost Inner Strength and Fitness

Everyone consumes food to develop and keep a sound body, yet we all have different dietary requirements as babies, kids, teens, young adults, and seniors. For instance, newborns require food at a specific time every day until they reach a specific age and can eat more satiating food varieties to eventually eat three times daily. In any case, as most guardians know, kids and young adults often snack between meals. Seniors also habitually snack, so it is fair to say that snacking isn't restricted to any age.

There are healthy and unhealthy food sources among the limitless number of food varieties you can put in your body, and it is critical to avoid the wrong food sources whenever possible. While many people are good at avoiding bad food sources, selecting the absolute best food sources for their nutritional goals is much more difficult. We are here to make it easier for you to find the most elite food, Power Foods. Check out the accompanying detailed breakdown for some of my top picks.

- **Beef**

This kind of meat is a great choice due to its high good cholesterol, protein content, and saturated fat that support a healthy body by increasing levels of energy and testosterone. Naturally raised dairy cattle are a better source of beef since they are primarily grass-fed rather than grain-fed and their meat contains significantly more omega-3 unsaturated fats and conjugated linoleic acid (CLA). CLA, a solid fat found in beef, has been shown in preliminary trials to help reduce body fat while supporting muscle and strength growth.

- **Salmon**

Salmon is high in omega-3 unsaturated fats, DHA (docosahexaenoic acid that is required to maintain and enhance normal brain function), and EPA (eicosapentaenoic acids that positively affect coronary heart disease, inflammation, and hypertension). According to a review, people who consumed more omega-3 had better muscle strength and insulin sensitivity which increases muscle protein blend (muscle development) and increases amino acid and glucose absorption.

- **Eggs**

The ideal source of protein, eggs, come with HDL (good) cholesterol and are ordinarily considered a bad food choice, yet that couldn't be farther from the truth as they are filled with several benefits. For example, eggs help with keeping up testosterone levels and muscle lining. In one review, subjects who ate three eggs a day while following a yoga program increased their muscle size and strength twice as much as those who consumed only one egg or no eggs a day. In investigations, 640 milligrams a day of good cholesterol from eggs diminished LDL (bad) cholesterol in the body.

- **Herring**

Herring is wealthy in omega-3s and probably has the highest creatine content, which can assist with helping muscle strength and development, of any food source.

- **Brown rice**

Brown rice is a whole grain that is filled with fiber to assist in bowel movement and keep insulin levels consistent, providing individuals with steady energy throughout the day. In addition, it has large quantities of gamma-aminobutyric, an amino acid that fills in as a synapse for the cells in the body and supports chemical reactions.

- **Wheat**

Wheat is plentiful in iron, zinc, potassium, selenium, and B nutrients and high in protein with many expanded chain amino acids, arginine, and glutamine. Moreover, it is high in fiber, making it an extraordinary source of slow-processing sugars. It has an abundance of octacosanol which supports exercises and workouts and can increase muscle strength and perseverance.

- **Bread**

Bread made from natural grains like millet, wheat, spelt, and oat, and from vegetables, for example, lentils or soybeans is a good food source as it is high in protein and has every one of the nine amino acids your body needs for muscle development. Moreover, these whole grains and vegetables digest slowly, increasing fat consumption over the day and providing more energy for exercise.

- **Spinach**

Spinach not just enhances well-being through its rich inventory of cancer prevention agents, but also develops muscle strength and size. It is an incredible source of glutamine which is profoundly significant for the immune system, brain function, and gut health. Spinach is also known to increase growth hormone levels and metabolic rate.

- **Yoga diet fundamentals**

If you have any desire to follow a yoga diet, you ought to eat as indicated by the standards recorded beneath:

- *Consistently consume the six Rasas, or tastes, which include sweet, pungent, salty, bitter, sour, and astringent flavors.*
- *Sweet-tasting food varieties such as cereals, dairy, wheat, dates, and rice should be eaten first during meals as these take longer to digest and are dense in nature.*
- *Then, move on to foods that are salty or sour tasting.*
- *Wrap up the meals with food types that are pungent (like peppers or onions), astringent (like tea or green apples), and bitter (like kale, celery, or green vegetables).*
- *Eat slowly and abstain from talking, giggling, and any other interruptions.*
- *Wait at least 3 hours between meals and try not to go over six hours without eating.*
- *Focus on breakfast and lunch. Numerous Ayurvedic specialists and yogis advocate for a light breakfast and a filling lunch. Supper might be consumed based on your hunger levels.*

- **Yoga diet fundamentals for special cases**

  - *Diabetes patients should follow the above proposals and take care of their glucose levels; attempt to keep everyday glucose levels as near to normal as expected.*

  - *Individuals with sporadic daily work routines ought to attempt to adhere to a dinner, lunch, and breakfast routine with little nibbling in between.*

  - *People who need to get in shape ought to avoid sweet and greasy food sources and generally eat fruits, vegetables, and nuts, with a decrease in dairy and meat products.*

Conclusion

Most people think of yoga as an activity involving only the physical body, but yoga is much more than that. Yoga is the art of moving through life in a psychological, emotional, and physical way. It aids in achieving solidity and consideration in the awareness of one's internal identity and learning about the mind, feelings, and actual necessities, as well as how to adapt to life's difficulties. Regular yoga practice results in positive body change, such as strong muscles, flexibility, adaptability, tolerance, and a sense of well-being. Best of all, you do not have to wait another day to get your life all set and disease-free; you can start practicing yoga today!

Yoga is considered somewhat basic because of its simplicity, but many people are unaware of its benefits in uniting the body, mind, and emotions for people from any age group, with any body type or size, and physical well-being and fitness level. Anyone can start practicing yoga and adapt different Asanas as per their needs.

Through this book, you have explored the simplest path to achieving health and peace and changing your life into the one you dream about. While this book is overwhelmingly dedicated to seniors, it can be used by individuals from any age group due to its versatile and entirely safe Asanas covering a range of different issues and end goals. You do not have to worry about what you need to do to fix your back pains or any other physical problem anymore. Just simply use _**Yoga for Seniors Ages 50-70**_ to create a regular yoga routine that will help you to shed your body's physical and mental stress. So, start practicing yoga today but remember to move in moderation, and you are good! Follow the guidelines mentioned in this book and try to understand the theories behind the different poses to help your body master them in a few weeks. I am sure you will find all the required information about yoga in this book.

I hope you enjoyed this book. I have tried my best to add all my knowledge regarding yoga and its different poses into this book. I advise you as a well-wisher to start believing in yourself and have faith in your abilities in every aspect of your life. Your life will begin progressing in the right direction as soon you start having confidence and belief in yourself. So, in the end, I wish you the best of luck in your life ahead. Stay happy, and always love your body first!

Thank you once again for purchasing this book and we hope you found it useful. Please consider leaving an honest review online check out some of our other publications using the link below:

thestarpublications.com

Visit the link below to grab your free gift:

thestarpublications.com/#get-a-free-book

If you have any **query**, please feel free to write us at:

info@thestarpublications.com

Made in the USA
Middletown, DE
06 October 2024

62079298R00080